BREATHE

Stop Overthinking, Calm Your Emotions &
Change Your Life

Author: Kate Simpson

Illustration: Joellen McCosh

Design: Diane Dempsey Murray

breathe-journal.com

Copyright © Take Two Consulting, LLC

DBA The BREATHE Journal

ISBN: 979-8-218-43298-0

BREATHE

Stop Overthinking, Calm Your Emotions &
Change Your Life

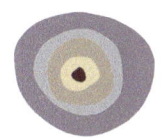

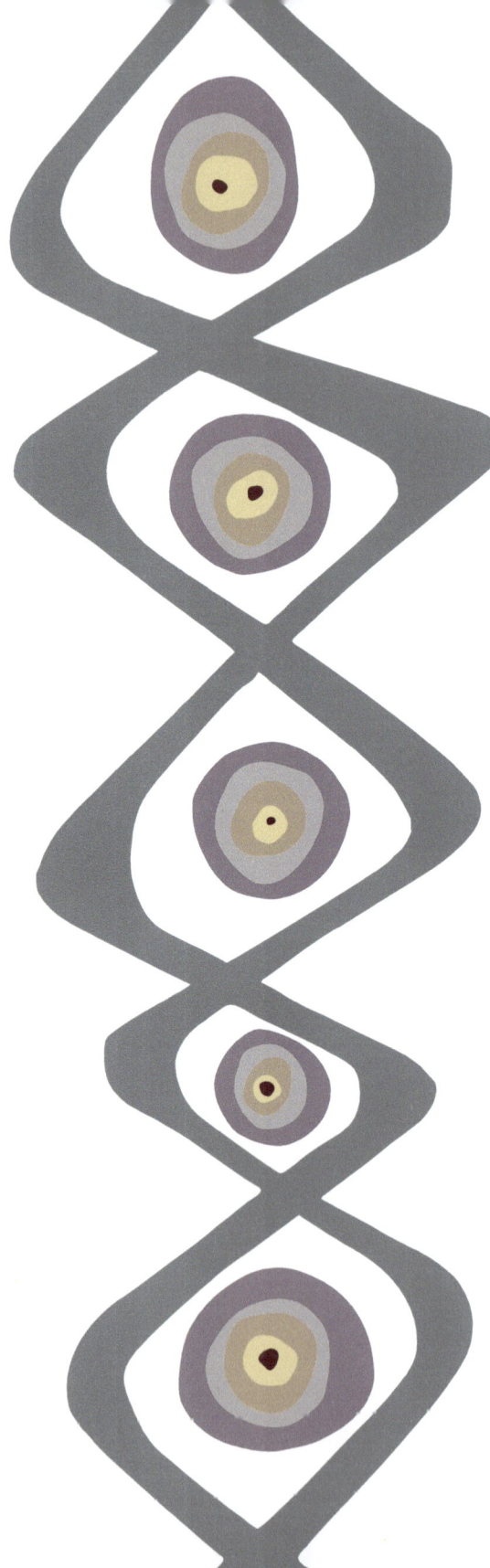

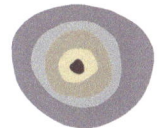

I'm dedicated to making positive changes in my life.

I know that it will take work, practice, and perseverance, but I'm worth the effort!

_____

NAME

_____

DATE

See BREATHE's website for free downloads and resources:

breathe-journal.com

Table of Contents

Begin Your Journey Here

IF YOU'RE READING THIS, chances are you're looking to make a change in your life. Maybe you're struggling with overthinking and seeking freedom from your thoughts. Perhaps you've gone through a significant transition—a breakup, a loss, or simply feel that something needs to shift.

No matter why you arrived here—you're welcome. Think of this space as your refuge, where you can slow down and begin the important work of self-reflection. It's a chance to uncover what's been holding you back from moving forward.

This journal is unlike others you might have encountered—it offers a practical roadmap to guide you through a unique self-exploration process. The practices offered here are backed by cutting-edge psychology. But more importantly, they've been successfully used by thousands of people to create real improvements in their lives. The journal will lead you through a 4-stage journey, exploring various aspects of yourself and your life. By the end, you'll have a clear idea of where you want to go, what's holding you back, and a set of tools to support you on your new path.

Using the changing seasons as a guide, you'll start your journey in **Stage 1: Winter**. Here, you'll slow down, observe, and reflect on the thoughts that shape your emotions. How do they influence your actions? You'll be encouraged to pause and notice that there's freedom in the space between your thoughts and actions—an opportunity to make new choices. You'll finish the section by showing yourself compassion for past choices driven by unexamined thoughts and recognize you were simply doing your best.

In Stage 2: Spring, you'll reflect on what you'd like to "grow" in your life through a guided "Ideal Day" meditation and exercises to uncover your values and assess if your life currently aligns with them. You'll then explore any limiting beliefs you hold that may impact what you think you're capable of and turn them into empowering, positive affirmations to release their hold over your thinking. You'll also spend time uncovering the origin of those limiting beliefs—most likely from your childhood.

In Stage 3: Summer, your focus shifts to your external world and the people around you. Do they reflect the life you envision for yourself? Are they supportive of the person you want to become? If they don't, how do you cultivate a new community? You'll also explore the important concept of boundaries—learning how to establish and communicate them. Towards the end of this stage, you'll practice reconnecting by offering others simple kindnesses, acknowledging the universal experience of emotional suffering, and ultimately extending compassion to those who have hurt you—a critical component of fostering your well-being.

In Stage 4: Autumn, the final phase, you'll cultivate an appreciation for the bounty of your work by training your thoughts to notice the positives in your life. By this stage, regardless of whether you find it easy or challenging to find things to be grateful for, you'll have completed reflective exercises and deserve to reap the benefits of your hard work. As you examine your life during the 30-day gratitude practice, you'll discover much to be thankful for.

Each stage, each "season" of this journey, is like a crucial stepping stone. When you follow along, each step provides a clear path across the turbulent river of change. It's hard but life-changing work. How long will it take? The answer depends on how much you truly desire change. It won't happen without a commitment.

The exercises in this journal will open the door to a life filled with greater contentment and abundance. This is an invitation to step through. **What awaits on the other side? The ability to simply BREATHE.**

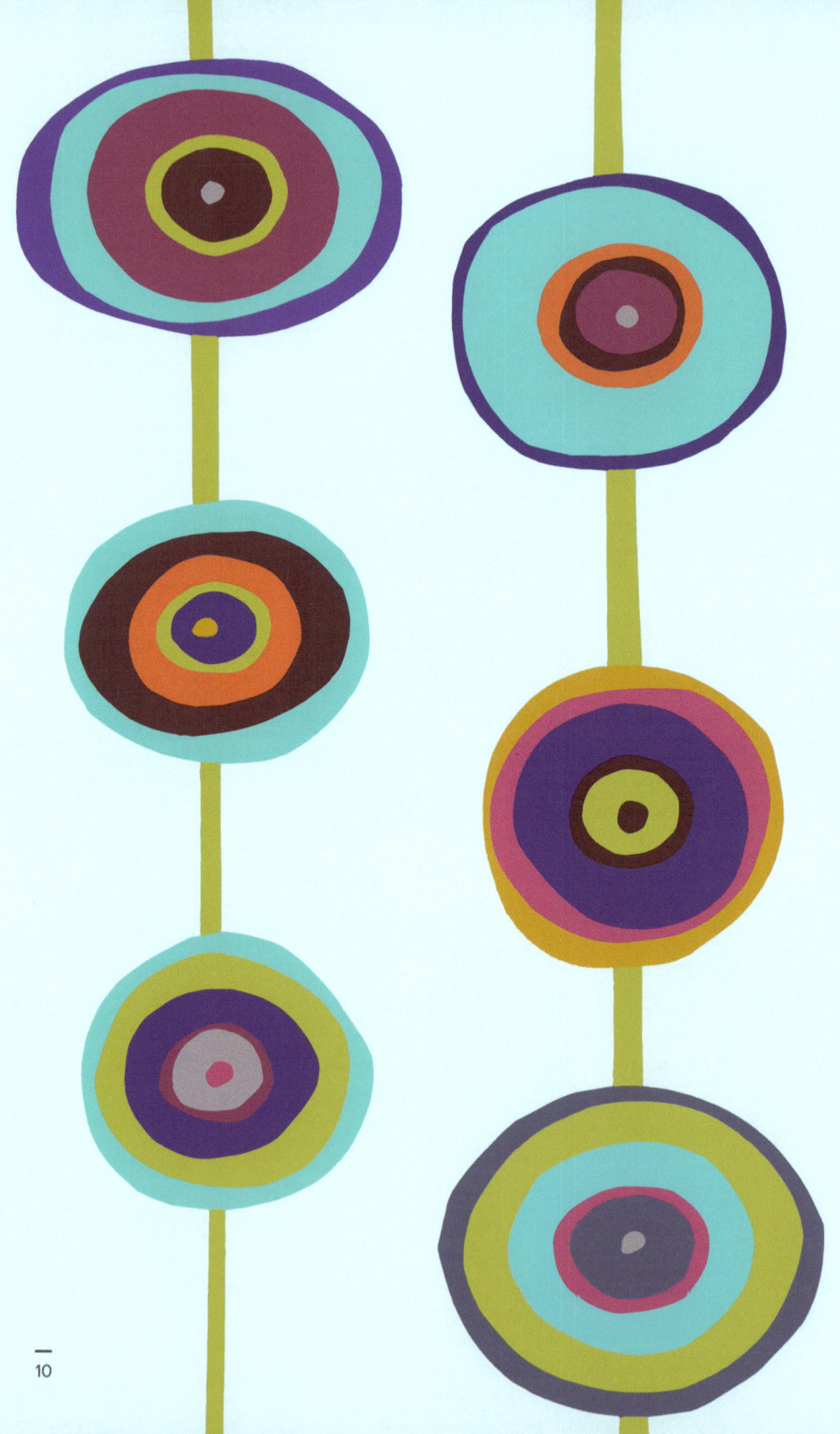

WINTER

EXPLORING YOUR THOUGHTS

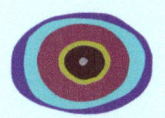

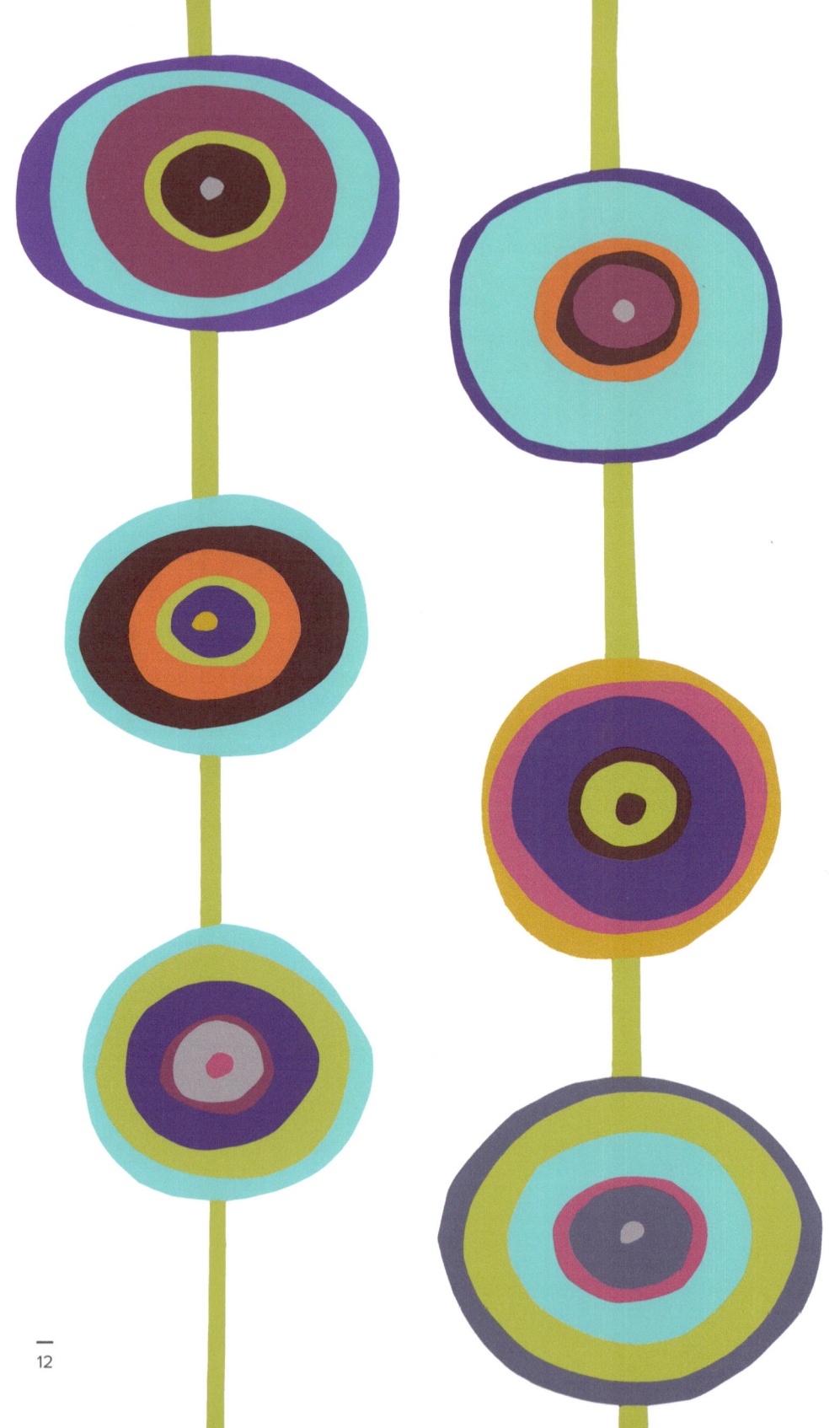

Exploring Your Thoughts

The winter season, characterized by less daylight, long nights, and quiet stillness, serves as the perfect metaphor for the work you're going to do in this section. Self-reflection and self-discovery require work similar to wintertime's slow but steady perseverance. While it may feel uncomfortable, this inner work is critical to reemerge in a new way in the springtime. Just as the natural world needs winter hibernation for its spring bloom, you, too, need to engage in a period of inner renewal. These practices lay the foundation for the possibility of something new and better, but only if you first give yourself the gift of wintering.

Welcome to the Winter Stage.

Meditation demystified

You've heard the term before. Maybe you've even read about meditation's benefits because there are many, both for your physical and emotional health. Scientific studies show that just 10 minutes of meditation each day for eight weeks can significantly improve your brain's "neuroplasticity" (i.e., flexibility), which has been linked to greater emotional regulation and feelings of calm, less attachment to thoughts (rumination), and fewer feelings of anxiety and depression. But you may still be wondering: "Why should I make time for meditation? And how would I get started?"

In a nutshell, meditation is a way to train your awareness to notice your thoughts so they don't control your actions. An easy way to understand it is to picture your thoughts as a river—sometimes wild, sometimes calm, but always flowing. When your thoughts are wild, it's easy to get swept away by them. You might get so caught up that you don't even realize you're in turbulent waters. You're just desperately trying to stay afloat. And when this happens, you lose control over how you respond to your thoughts.

Meditation trains your awareness to recognize the flow of the river. Once you gain that awareness, you can step out of it, regardless of how intense the emotions or thoughts may be. A meditation practice strengthens the capacity to observe your thoughts, reducing the likelihood of being swept away into reactivity. Once outside of the river, you have the opportunity to observe, notice, and be curious about the condition of the water (i.e., your thoughts). Is it rushing? Is it calm?

Learning to observe your mind isn't easy. Think of it like a muscle that you've barely used before. Just as you need to train any muscle with regular trips to the gym, training your awareness to notice your thoughts requires consistent, regular practice. While trying it once won't hurt, you won't see any significant improvements in how you feel without regular practice. Remember, even 10 minutes a day can change the architecture of your mind.

The power of observing your thoughts

Stepping out of that rushing water presents new opportunities in your life. While this may sound like an exaggeration, consider this: when you pause before reacting, taking note of your thoughts and emotions rather than being swept away by them, you open the door to different outcomes. You gain the freedom to choose how you respond to a situation.

Think of a scenario that usually creates an emotional reaction for you. For example, when someone says something hurtful or triggering, your immediate response might be to speak harshly to them, cut off contact, or silently feel angry. While these habitual reactions are understandable, they also lead to a well-worn outcome. But what if you chose to respond differently?

Instead of reacting without conscious awareness, you can choose to approach the situation with curiosity. Perhaps something is troubling the other person; maybe they received bad news, are feeling overwhelmed in their lives, or are generally struggling. If you could entertain alternative explanations for their behavior, would you respond differently?

Let's say you choose to respond with curiosity. In a calm and grounded way, you reach out to them and express how their actions affected you, using "I statements" (which you'll learn in Stage 3). You tell them you're concerned about them and ask if they're okay. Maybe you discover that they're dealing with a significant challenge. They may apologize and open up about what they're experiencing. You've created a new outcome—improved communication and a deeper connection. This is big! You've created a different path because of your newfound awareness of your thoughts, pausing, and choosing not to react to them.

Of course, your friend might respond defensively or blame you for their reaction. This is important information for you to objectively notice and decide how you'd like to respond. Perhaps they're not the friend you thought they were and, instead, someone trapped in their thoughts and emotions. Now, you can consciously choose whether you'd like to deepen, maintain, or distance the connection, or perhaps let the relationship go.

As you train your mind not to react to your thoughts, you gain more power to choose how you respond to every situation and create the opportunity for different and possibly better outcomes.

How to start meditating

Set your phone timer for 10 minutes. Sit upright, close your eyes, and focus on your breath. Notice your chest rising as you inhale slowly, then exhale. Soon, your mind will wander into a variety of thoughts: important decisions, concerns, or tasks on your to-do list, even external sensations. This is normal! Even experienced meditators encounter a stream of thoughts. When a thought arises, silently acknowledge it with "Thinking," then return your focus to your breath.

Repeat this process throughout the 10 minutes: acknowledge the thought with "Thinking," then breathe.

Continue this practice whenever you notice you've drifted away in thought. This repetition trains your mind to "wake up" from the trance of thinking. Though it may feel frustrating, remember that the ability to break away from your thoughts offers a chance to change: you'll gain the freedom to attend to your thoughts in new ways.

ACTION STEP   Experience meditation

If you're finding it challenging to begin (perhaps your thoughts feel overwhelming or you're too distracted), this guided meditation will gently walk you through the experience.

All meditations can be found at:
breathe-journal.com/meditations

PROMPT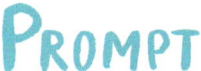

Reflecting on your meditation experience

During your meditation today, what thoughts or emotions came up for you? Were there any surprises? How did you find the experience overall? Was it more difficult or easier than you anticipated?

Prompt

Reflecting on your meditation experience (continued)

A two-week meditation challenge

You've learned about the benefits of regular meditation practice: by strengthening your ability to distance yourself from your thoughts, you can respond to situations with awareness rather than "mindlessness," a term coined by Harvard professor Ellen Langer.

Try it for the next two weeks—commit to meditating for just 10 minutes each day. When you think: "I don't have the time," consider how much time you spend on your phone each day, and then question if it's true. The quiet of the morning, before anyone else is awake, or in the evening, just before bed, tends to work best for most people. Set your phone on silent, use its timer, or explore a free meditation app like Insight Timer, which tracks your total meditation time.

Try it for the next two weeks— commit to meditating for just 10 minutes each day.

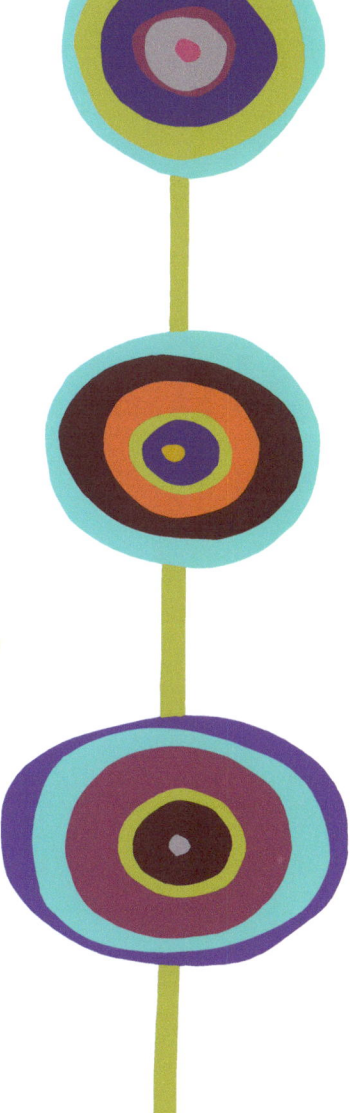

Navigating intense emotions

THE ABILITY TO CREATE SPACE from strong emotions, not to be swept up into unconscious reactivity, but to observe the feelings, let yourself experience them, and ultimately let them pass is critical to your ability to overcome and move forward towards something new and better. As Susan David, a Harvard-based psychologist and author of *Emotional Agility* says, "When you can just be with your emotions, your gentle acceptance defangs that difficulty or challenge a little bit, allowing you to take the next brave step towards what matters most."

This next process is a helpful technique for creating distance

PROMPT

STEP 1

Exploring a challenging situation

Consider a situation that triggers challenging emotions. It could be why you picked up this journal—perhaps there's a part of your life that needs to change. Is there a painful situation or challenge happening for you now or that happened in the past? Do you have a specific fear about the future that keeps you awake at night? Have you experienced a difficult transition or loss?

Write about this situation here. Take your time. If you don't have the time to finish it now, come back later. This is your process, and there's no set schedule.

from intense emotions, called Emotionally Expressive Journaling. It's a simple three-step process that helps you create mental space when writing about something challenging. As you're learning, any technique that enables you to distance yourself from your thoughts and feelings can be helpful because it allows you to respond to them differently. This is the key to charting a better path forward.

You can return to this section and use this technique whenever necessary. It can be used with any difficult situation or relationship in your life when you need some help creating space from intense emotions.

PROMPT

Exploring a challenging situation (continued)

Identify your feelings

Now, listen to the guided meditation. Then, go back and read through your story as if you were a neutral observer. What difficult emotions do you notice? You might find some feelings in your writing, such as hurt, frustration, insecurity, anger, fear, or sadness.

Identify your emotions

Put a check mark next to each emotion you identify in your story

SADNESS

Ashamed	Grieving	Lonely	Rejected
Betrayed	Hopeless	Lost	Unmotivated
Depressed	Hurt	Miserable	Weak
Disappointed	Isolated	Neglected	Worthless

FEAR

Anxious	Panic	Shock	Trapped
Confused	Paranoid	Stress	Uncomfortable
Insecure	Scared	Suspicious	
Nervous	Self-conscious	Tense	
Overwhelmed	Skeptical	Terrified	

ANGER

Aggravated	Disgust	Furious	Irritated
Aggressive	Envious	Grumpy	Jealous
Annoyed	Foolish	Hateful	Rage
Bitter	Frustrated	Hostile	Resentful

PROMPT

Write down each emotion you find or
notice in your challenging situation

Review the list of emotions you've written down. The simple act of putting them on paper begins to create distance from them. Perhaps you've already noticed a slight decrease in their intensity? Now, let's try a technique from Acceptance and Commitment Therapy (ACT), known to further deepen this sense of separation:

For each emotion you've listed, quietly say the following to yourself:

"I notice that I'm feeling (insert identified emotion)."

Afterward, tune into the sensations in your body. Take a deep breath and focus your attention there. Sit with the sensations for a moment. Although this might feel challenging, emotions can reside in the body without you knowing. And unacknowledged emotions dormant in the body can negatively impact your physical health.

You can practice this exercise anytime you experience a challenging emotion. Your awareness of your emotional experiences will grow with continued meditation practice. Throughout your day, use this technique: "I notice that I'm feeling _____ ."

For instance, if your partner or family member does something hurtful, and you start to feel angry, upset, sad, or anxious, quietly say to yourself, "I notice that I'm feeling _____." Next, BREATHE. Allow yourself to experience the sensation fully in your body. Observe any resistance to that feeling and try to soften and release it. Notice if the emotion becomes less overwhelming as you create space from it. Within this space, you can consciously choose how you want to respond to the situation rather than reacting with "mindlessness."

ACTION STEP Mindful body awareness

Emotions often manifest and settle into the body, sometimes before the mind notices them. Ignored emotions can lead to physical issues over time, so it's important to pay attention and recognize what you're feeling and where. Try this body scan meditation to focus on the different parts of your body and identify any tension or stress it may be holding.

Return to this body scan meditation whenever you're experiencing difficult emotions, stress, or anxiety.

It's important to pay attention and recognize what you're feeling and where.

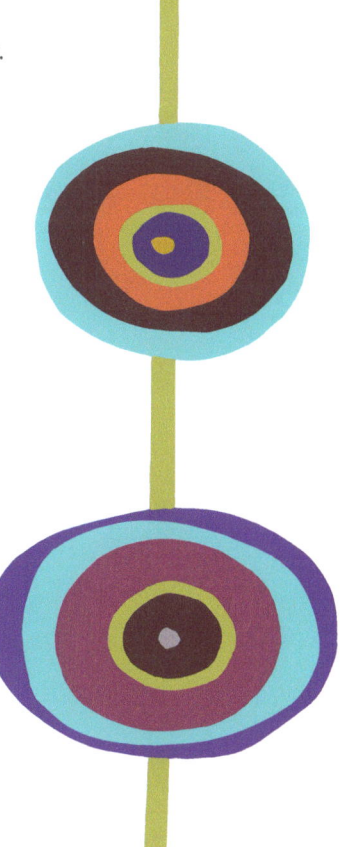

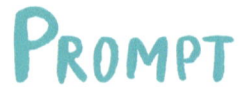

PROMPT

Gaining perspective

This prompt is crucial for your journey and moving forward in a positive direction. Although it's challenging, taking the time to reflect on a painful situation, and seeing it in the broader context of your life, can be incredibly beneficial.

If you're still experiencing grief from the situation you wrote about, check out "The Five Stages of Grief" (from the book *On Death and Dying* by psychologist Elisabeth Kübler-Ross) to learn more about this natural but nonlinear journey. Remember, there's no set timeline for healing. If you find the prompt below difficult to answer right now, that's okay. You can return to this prompt whenever you feel ready.

Reflect on how the situation you described fits into the bigger picture of your life. Write about whether this experience has changed how you value certain aspects of your life and if you now see this situation in a new light.

The importance of self-kindness

AS YOU START TO OBSERVE your thoughts more closely, you may notice how many of them are unkind when directed at yourself. In the next section, you'll explore limiting beliefs and self-judgment, but it's crucial not to believe those negative thoughts. One way to do this is by offering yourself kindness and compassion, which leads to greater self-acceptance. Just as nurturing and self-care are vital for the natural

ACTION STEP   Practice kindness to yourself

Take a moment to consider activities that bring you happiness or contentment, times when worries of the day fade away and time seems to stand still. It could be reading a good book, walking in nature, connecting with a good friend, getting a massage, enjoying your favorite music, cooking a favorite meal, or engaging in a creative activity.

List five things you'll do for yourself over the next week:

1. _____

2. _____

3. _____

4. _____

5. _____

Schedule each activity into your day or week, treating them with the same importance as any other task. After completing each one, cross it off.

world to regenerate during the winter season, prioritizing your well-being is essential for replenishing your energy. Have you noticed that self-care often ends up at the bottom of your to-do list? Yet isn't your own well-being just as deserving of attention as others in your life?

In these following exercises, you'll have the opportunity to practice self-care and cultivate self-compassion.

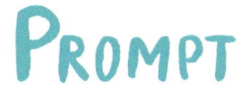

PROMPT

Reflecting on self-care

How does it feel to take time for yourself? Do you experience feelings of guilt, happiness, relief, stress, or something else?

Practicing self-compassion

AS YOU BECOME MORE AWARE of your thoughts and emotions, you may notice some of them as self-critical or self-judgmental. These familiar patterns of self-blame often stem from childhood messages, which you'll explore further in the next section. When was the last time you showed yourself kindness after making a mistake? Aren't you doing your best given everything happening in your life right now? Don't you deserve the same understanding and compassion you'd offer a friend in a similar situation?

These exercises will help you cultivate self-compassion and extend grace to yourself.

ACTION STEP   Guided meditation for self-compassion

 Sometimes, it's tough to be kind to ourselves. This guided meditation can help show you how to offer compassion to yourself. Give it a try and see how it feels.

When was the last time you showed yourself kindness after making a mistake?

PROMPT

Finding compassion for your younger self

Imagine yourself as a child. You can either find a photo of your younger self or simply close your eyes and visualize. Picture that small, vulnerable, innocent, and trusting version of you. Reflect on the ups and downs they'll face—the struggles, joys, insecurities, and sorrows. What gentle and empathetic advice would you offer to that younger version of yourself? Write it down here.

PROMPT

Finding compassion for your younger self (continued)

PROMPT

**Writing a compassionate
letter to yourself**

Fast forward to the future and envision an older, wiser,
nonjudgmental, and unconditionally loving version of yourself.
This future self has experienced all the highs and lows you've
gone through and has gained profound wisdom and empathy.
Imagine this version of you looking back on your current life.
What words of encouragement, understanding, and compassion
would they offer you now? Write a letter from your future self to
your present self, offering guidance and support.

Dear Me,

[Your compassionate letter here]

With much love,
Your older self

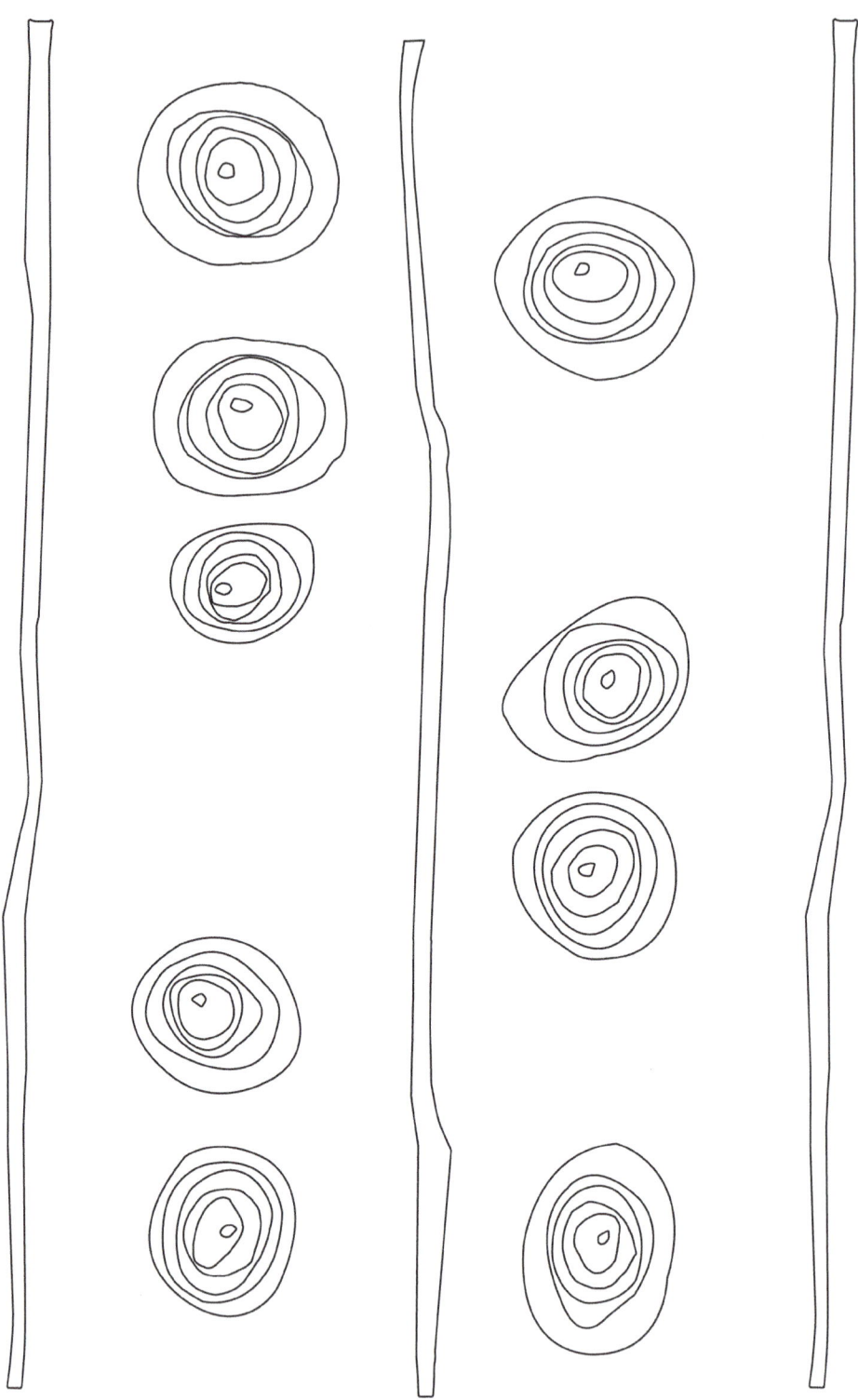

Color to calm your mind and stop overthinking

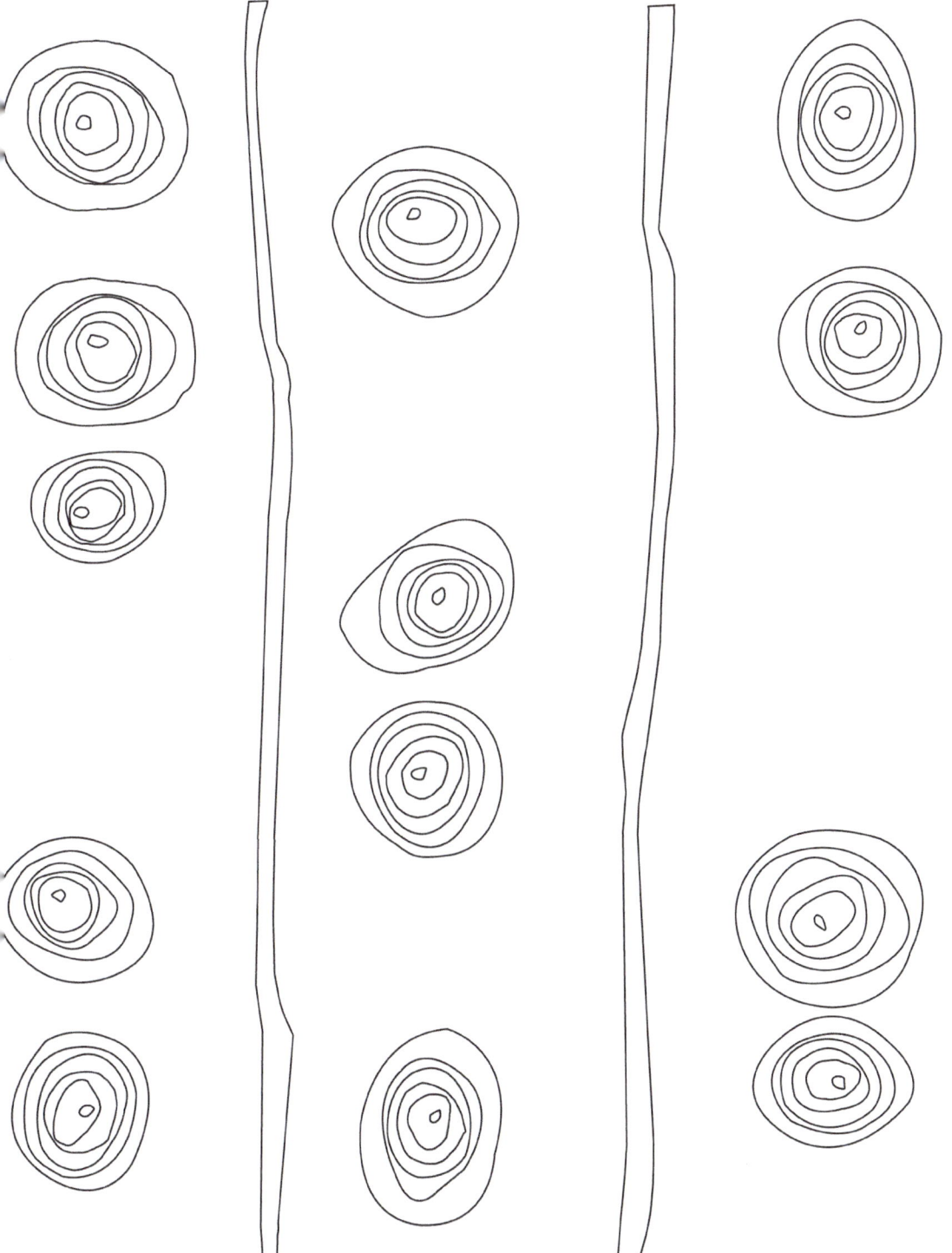

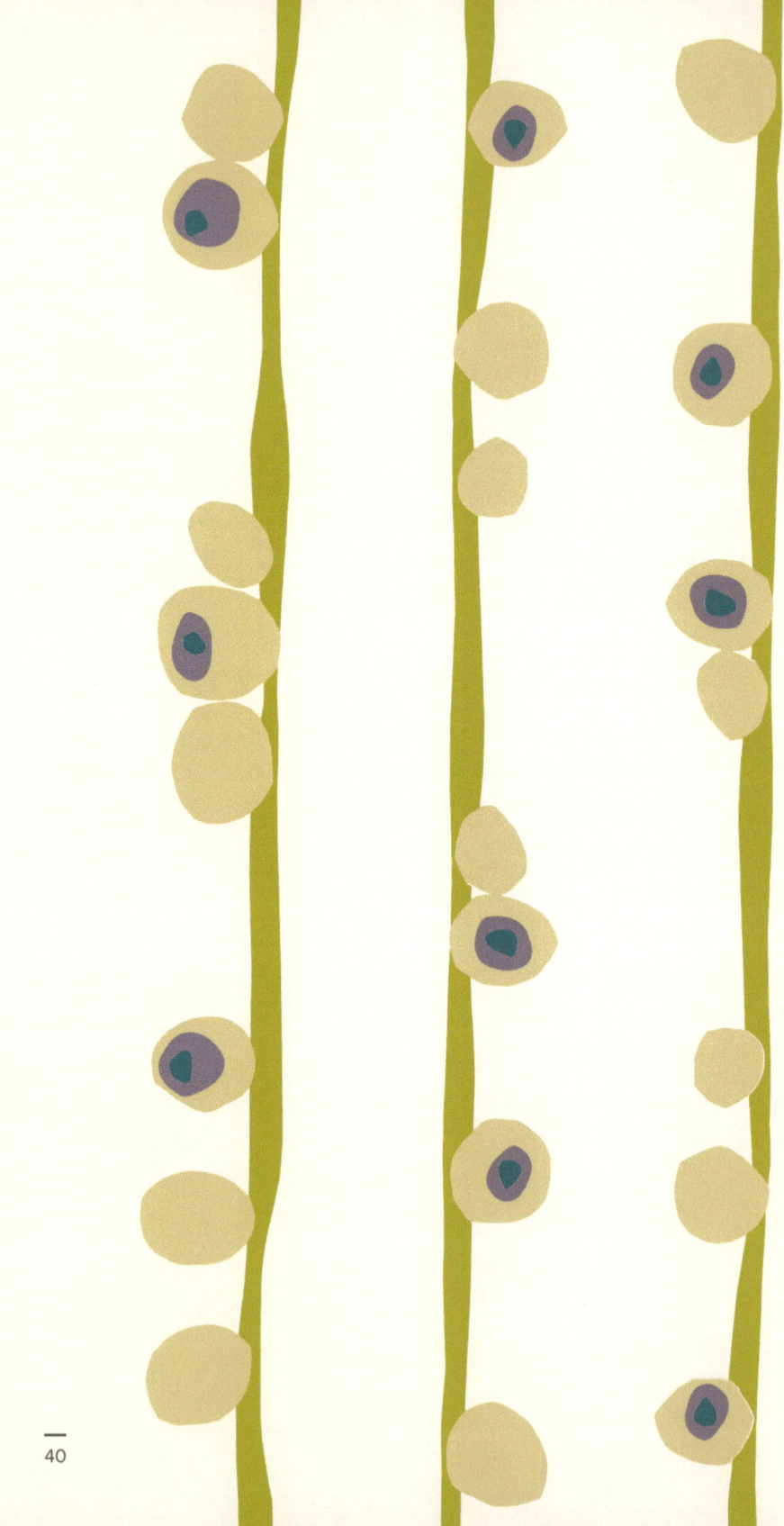

SPRING

CHARTING A NEW PATH

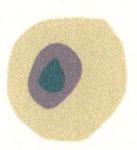

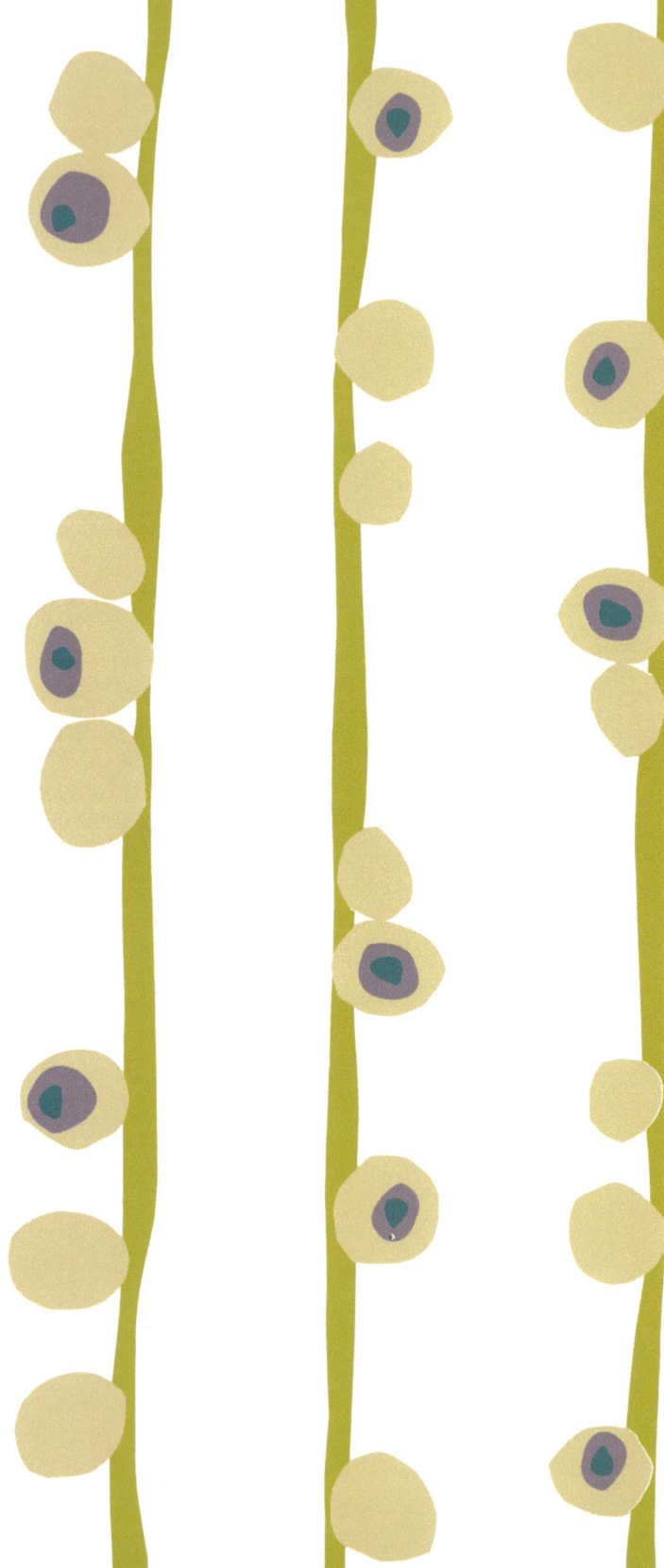

Charting a New Path

Springtime. The season of renewal and emergence from the darkness of winter. As you emerge from the dark, cocoon-like self-reflection work of winter into the brighter days of spring, you'll have a deeper understanding of your thoughts and a greater capacity to offer yourself compassion. You can now direct your attention to your desires, aspirations, and goals for the future. You arrived at BREATHE seeking change. This stage allows you to explore the metaphorical seeds you'd like to plant and identify any self-limiting beliefs that may hurt their growth.

What do you desire?

WHEN WAS THE LAST TIME YOU spent time reflecting on what truly matters to you and what your ideal life looks like? You may be tempted to jump right into action, but, just as it's essential to consult a map before starting a journey, it's crucial to have a clear direction to avoid getting lost on the way. Whether it's about relationships, work, or life in general, giving yourself this reflective time will ensure that you make choices that align with your values.

In the following exercises, you'll explore your desires through three steps. First, you'll envision your ideal day via a guided meditation. Next, you'll examine your core values. Finally, you'll assess your current life to see how well it aligns with your vision and outline practical steps for necessary change.

ACTION STEP Guided meditation for your ideal day

Take a moment to listen to this guided meditation designed to lead you through your ideal day.

PROMPT

Describing your ideal day

Write about your ideal day from morning to night. Be detailed, describe how the day looks and feels, and be specific. Include where you are when you wake up, who you spend time with, and what activities fill your day. Capture the emotions and sensations you'd like to experience.

PROMPT

Describing your ideal day (continued)

Identifying your values

UNDERSTANDING YOUR VALUES is crucial for making decisions that align with your true self. Without clarity of your values, you may feel uneasy or dissatisfied without understanding why. Take a minute to reflect on moments when you felt most aligned with your values and times when you felt out of sync.

As you look through the list of values, which five resonate most strongly with you? Circle each one.

Acceptance	Determination	Independence	Reliability
Accountability	Diversity	Inner harmony	Reputation
Achievement	Do good work	Innovation	Respect
Adventure	Duty	Integrity	Responsibility
Authenticity	Egalitarianism	Justice	Safety
Authority	Empathy	Kindness	Security
Autonomy	Fairness	Knowledge	Self-respect
Balance	Faith	Leadership	Sensitivity
Beauty	Family	Learning	Service
Boldness	Flexibility	Listening	Solidarity
Bravery	Friendship	Love	Spirituality
Compassion	Fun	Loyalty	Stability
Challenge	Generosity	Mastery	Status
Collaboration	Gratitude	Openness	Success
Community	Growth	Opportunity	Sustainability
Competency	Happiness	Optimism	Transparency
Contribution	Hard work	Patience	Trustworthiness
Courage	Helping	Peace	Vulnerability
Creativity	Honesty	Perseverance	Willingness
Curiosity	Humility	Punctuality	Wisdom
Dependability	Humor	Recognition	
	Inclusion	Reconciliation	

Prompt

Reflecting on your values

Recall a time when you felt like you were living **in alignment** with your values. Describe the situation and the choices you made. How did you feel during that phase in your life? Which values were reflected? Use the list of values at the left to help.

PROMPT

Reflecting on your values (continued)

Now, think of a time when you were living **out of alignment**
with your values. Describe the choices you made.
How did you feel during that period in your life?
Which of your values were compromised?

PROMPT

Is your life aligned with what's important to you?

Now that you have a sense of what matters to you from reflecting on your ideal day and your core values, take a moment to evaluate how aligned your current life is with them. This exercise is like a snapshot, indicating your level of contentment and satisfaction in different areas of your life and showing you where you may need change.

Using the Wheel of Life below, place a dot in each area of your life to indicate your level of satisfaction. Then, connect the dots with a line. This visual representation will clearly illustrate your satisfaction levels across different areas of your life and help show you where you might direct energy for change. Think of it as a roadmap for enhancing your overall life contentment.

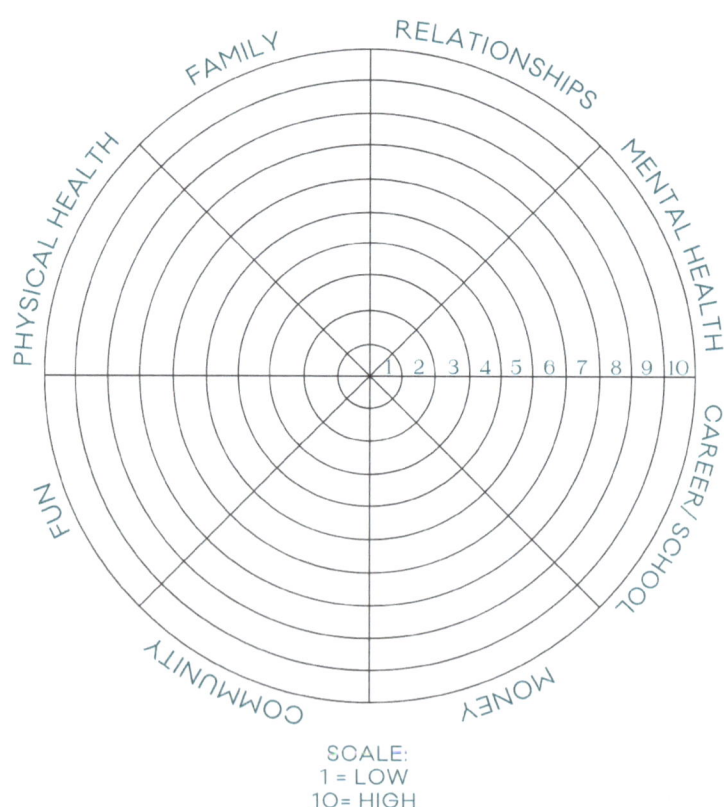

SCALE:
1 = LOW
10= HIGH

What does this exercise tell you about your life?

The change you seek

TAKE NOTE OF THE AREAS on your Wheel of Life where satisfaction levels are lower. Before change can happen, it's important to ask yourself, "What do I deeply desire?" As you think about this question, broaden your focus beyond narrow attachments to specific outcomes. If you find yourself saying,

"Once _____ happens, then I'll be happy,"

that's a sign to widen your lens. Instead, consider the desire underneath the attachment to the outcome. What are you truly longing for? These are the keys to finding greater contentment.

For example, you might believe you need a specific relationship to improve before you can feel "happy" or experience greater contentment. Look deeper: what's beneath your desire? Maybe you seek emotional intimacy, connection, or a sense of belonging. Perhaps you're hoping the outcome will prove what you struggle to believe: that you're worthy of love (you'll explore thoughts like this in the next section).

In each area of your life with a low score, write about how you could reach a "10," the highest level of satisfaction. Reflect on what you seek in each area in broader terms rather than fixating on specific outcomes.

RELATIONSHIPS

My deepest desire:

_____

_____

_____

MENTAL HEALTH

My deepest desire:

_____

_____

_____

CAREER/SCHOOL

My deepest desire:

_____

_____

_____

MONEY

My deepest desire:

_____

_____

_____

COMMUNITY

My deepest desire:

_____

_____

_____

FUN

My deepest desire:

_____

_____

_____

PHYSICAL HEALTH

My deepest desire:

_____

_____

_____

FAMILY

My deepest desire:

_____

_____

_____

Starting small

CHANGE OFTEN FEELS DAUNTING, like standing at the base of a huge mountain with it looming over you. Yet remember the wise phrase: "Even the longest journey begins with one step." Breaking down your desires into manageable actions can make achieving your goals less daunting.

As you think about your broader goals in different areas of your life and the changes needed to achieve them, what small steps can you take?

ACTION STEP   Take tiny steps

Choose a few areas of your life that scored a lower level of satisfaction and reread your deepest desire for them. Then, consider what small actions you can take today, next week, and next month to move closer to them. Remember to break them down into small, doable steps. These actions could include sending an e-mail, doing research, enrolling in a class, joining a new group, etc.

AREA OF MY LIFE REQUIRING CHANGE: _____

What I can do:

Today _____

Next Week _____

Next Month _____

AREA OF MY LIFE REQUIRING CHANGE: _____

What I can do:

Today _____

Next Week _____

Next Month _____

AREA OF MY LIFE REQUIRING CHANGE: _____

What I can do:

Today_____

Next Week _____

Next Month _____

AREA OF MY LIFE REQUIRING CHANGE: _____

What I can do:

Today_____

Next Week _____

Next Month _____

AREA OF MY LIFE REQUIRING CHANGE: _____

What I can do:

Today_____

Next Week _____

Next Month _____

AREA OF MY LIFE REQUIRING CHANGE: _____

What I can do:

Today_____

Next Week _____

Next Month _____

Repeat this process for any area of your life where change is needed.

Reshaping your mindset

YOU MAY START TO OBSERVE that specific thoughts recur frequently. It's common for the same thoughts to resurface (reportedly 95% of your thoughts repeat daily), and they're often rooted in negative beliefs about yourself (you're not good enough, smart enough, deserving enough). As these thoughts keep playing on repeat, they start feeling like truths. Believing these thoughts can influence what you think you can do, achieve, or deserve. They dictate your mindset, which acts like a lens and guides many of your actions and decisions.

Uncovering internal barriers to change

Consider the areas of your life where you don't have as much satisfaction and the steps you listed to make the changes needed to reach a "10" on your satisfaction scale. What thoughts arose? What's holding you back from taking the steps? While some goals have clear external barriers, others are more internal, crafted from your thoughts about what you believe you can achieve or deserve. As you've learned, thoughts are powerful, and when you believe them to be true, they shape the direction of your life.

Where do these "limiting beliefs" originate? As a child, you absorb the stories and messages about your value, lovability, intelligence, etc. Think about a negative message you received as a child. Do you notice similar messages in your thoughts about yourself now? It's like unearthing your roots to understand how you've grown into the person you are today.

Below are some common goals and the typical limiting beliefs that hold people back from achieving them.

GOAL: Finish school/get a new job/write a book

LIMITING BELIEF: I'm not (smart enough/skilled enough/creative enough) to accomplish my goal

....

GOAL: Get in better physical shape

LIMITING BELIEF: Taking care of myself means I'm selfish

....

GOAL: Have more time for myself by setting better boundaries when people ask me to do something for them

LIMITING BELIEF: I will let people down if I say "no"

....

GOAL: Find a new partner

LIMITING BELIEF: I don't deserve love

....

GOAL: Start a new business or project

LIMITING BELIEF: If I try something and fail, people will negatively judge me

....

GOAL: Find new friends

LIMITING BELIEF: People won't like me until I look a certain way

PROMPT

Identifying your goals and limiting beliefs

Write down three goals you'd like to achieve, and then identify a single limiting belief that may hold you back from achieving each one.

1. My goal: _____

Limiting belief: _____

_____

2. My goal:_____

Limiting belief: _____

_____

3. My goal:_____

Limiting belief: _____

_____

What other limiting beliefs may be holding you back?

Letting go of limiting beliefs

EXPLORING AND NAMING your limiting beliefs, and understanding where they originate, is helpful, but it won't free you from them. To accomplish that, you need to consciously replace them with new thoughts.

A powerful technique for replacing old beliefs is through positive affirmation work. Affirmations are constructive statements you repeat to yourself. Each time you repeat a thought, positive or negative, you deepen that thought pattern. Just like with meditation and training your mind to notice thoughts, affirmations require regular practice to be effective.

Affirmations are constructive statements you repeat to yourself.

The best way to use affirmations is to tailor them to your limiting beliefs. Let's revisit the examples from page 61:

LIMITING BELIEF: I'm not (smart enough/skilled enough/creative enough) to accomplish my goal

POSITIVE AFFIRMATION: I'm smart/skilled/creative enough to accomplish anything I set my mind to, and I have the power to change my life

....

LIMITING BELIEF: Taking care of myself means I'm selfish

POSITIVE AFFIRMATION: I prioritize my self-care because it's essential for my physical and emotional well-being

....

LIMITING BELIEF: I will let people down if I say "no"

POSITIVE AFFIRMATION: I prioritize my well-being by honoring my boundaries and respectfully saying "no" when necessary

....

LIMITING BELIEF: I don't deserve love

POSITIVE AFFIRMATION: I'm deserving of love and affection just as I am

....

LIMITING BELIEF: If I try something and fail, people will negatively judge me

POSITIVE AFFIRMATION: I'm confident in my abilities and understand that failure is a natural part of growth

....

LIMITING BELIEF: People won't like me until I look a certain way

POSITIVE AFFIRMATION: I'm worthy of love and acceptance just as I am and my value is not determined by my appearance

PROMPT

Transform your limiting beliefs

Convert each of your limiting beliefs
or self-judgments into positive affirmations.

1. Limiting belief: _____

Positive affirmation: _____

_____

2. Limiting belief: _____

Positive affirmation: _____

_____

3. Limiting belief: _____

Positive affirmation: _____

_____

Write down your positive affirmations on a sticky note and put them somewhere you'll see each day, like your bathroom mirror. Every time you notice the notes, say them either aloud or silently in your mind. Research suggests that saying them aloud in the morning while looking at yourself in the mirror can help your mind begin to believe them more quickly.

What other positive affirmations can you think of?

ACTION STEP   Integrate your positive affirmations

 Listen to this guided meditation to reinforce these positive affirmations in your mind by using an EMDR tapping technique that uses "bilateral stimulation" to allow your mind to more deeply integrate them.

Rewriting your childhood stories

AS YOU'VE DISCOVERED, your thoughts about what you can do, achieve, and have in your life are shaped by your limiting beliefs and self-judgments. They influence how you see yourself, the choices you've made in the past, and what you believe is possible in the future. How would your story change if you didn't believe them? How would it change if your limiting beliefs didn't affect your choices? In this exercise, you're going to imagine a new story, one free from limiting beliefs. You'll start by picking a limiting belief and explore how it has impacted your life. Then you'll reimagine what might have happened if, instead of accepting the limiting belief, you believed the inverse, the positive affirmation. A whole new world of possibilities will open up.

How would your life change if your limiting beliefs didn't affect your choices?

PROMPT

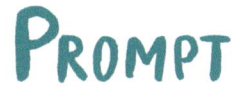

Shifting your narrative

Choose a limiting belief and its corresponding positive affirmation from your list. Holding the limiting belief in your mind, think about a specific aspect of your life that was affected by it—a particular situation, relationship, decision, action, etc. How did this belief affect the outcome?

EXAMPLES:

OLD STORY
**based on the limiting belief:
I'm unworthy of being loved**

"I used to believe that I wasn't good enough to have someone truly care about me. Because of this belief, I settled for relationships where I felt unloved and disrespected. I accepted people who treated me poorly, thinking it was all I deserved."

NEW STORY
**based on the positive affirmation:
I'm worthy of love**

"I now understand that I deserve love and respect in relationships. If I notice behavior that makes me feel unworthy or disrespected, I choose to walk away. I believe in my worth and refuse to settle for anything less than healthy, loving relationships."

OLD STORY
**based on the limiting belief:
I'm not good enough**

"I used to believe that I wasn't good enough to pursue my dream life. Because of this belief, I settled for situations that didn't fulfill me and made me feel trapped. I convinced myself I didn't have what it took to succeed."

NEW STORY
**based on the positive affirmation:
I'm capable**

"I now embrace my intelligence and potential. I recognize that my dreams are valid and achievable with dedication and effort. I'm taking steps towards my desired goals, confident in my abilities, and excited about the possibilities that lie ahead."

PROMPT

Shifting your narrative

Imagine how believing your positive affirmations would change your story. Write about the new possibilities that would open up for you.

Where did your limiting beliefs originate?

YOU WEREN'T BORN WITH SELF-JUDGMENTS and limiting beliefs. Most likely, they started with messages you received as a child, often from your family, caregivers, or your culture. The following exercise will help you begin to understand where they came from. This exercise is not about blaming your family, because—remember—they too had their own limiting beliefs from childhood. Instead, this prompt is designed to help you recognize that your limiting beliefs originated outside of you, despite how attached you may be to them. Knowing where they came from can help you let them go.

Knowing where limiting beliefs come from can help you let them go.

Prompt

Reflecting on your family

Think about your family of origin, and how they reacted in each of the scenarios below.

How did my family react when I . . .

Showed emotions like sadness or anger?

Didn't meet expectations or failed at something?

Acted differently from what was expected in my culture or society?

Had a conflict or disagreement with them?

Tried to be independent or make my own decisions?

As you think about each situation, pay attention to any negative reactions from your family. How did they communicate their expectations? Was their communication style clear, punitive, or passive-aggressive? What subtle or overt messages did you receive? Which of these messages did you internalize as your own beliefs?

Do you notice any similarities between the messages you received as a child and the limiting beliefs and self-judgments you now hold?

This exercise may be challenging, as family dynamics have many complex layers. Remember this is just the beginning. If you're working with a therapist, this exercise can serve as a valuable starting point for Family Systems Therapy, also known as "part work," where you explore and heal the parts of yourself that were wounded as a child and continue to influence your decisions today.

PROMPT

Reflecting on your family

How did your family react when you
showed emotions like sadness or anger?

How did your family react when you didn't meet expectations or failed at something?

Prompt

Reflecting on your family

How did your family react when you acted differently from what was expected in your culture or society?

How did your family react when you had a
conflict or disagreement with them?

How did your family react when you tried to be
independent or make your own decisions?

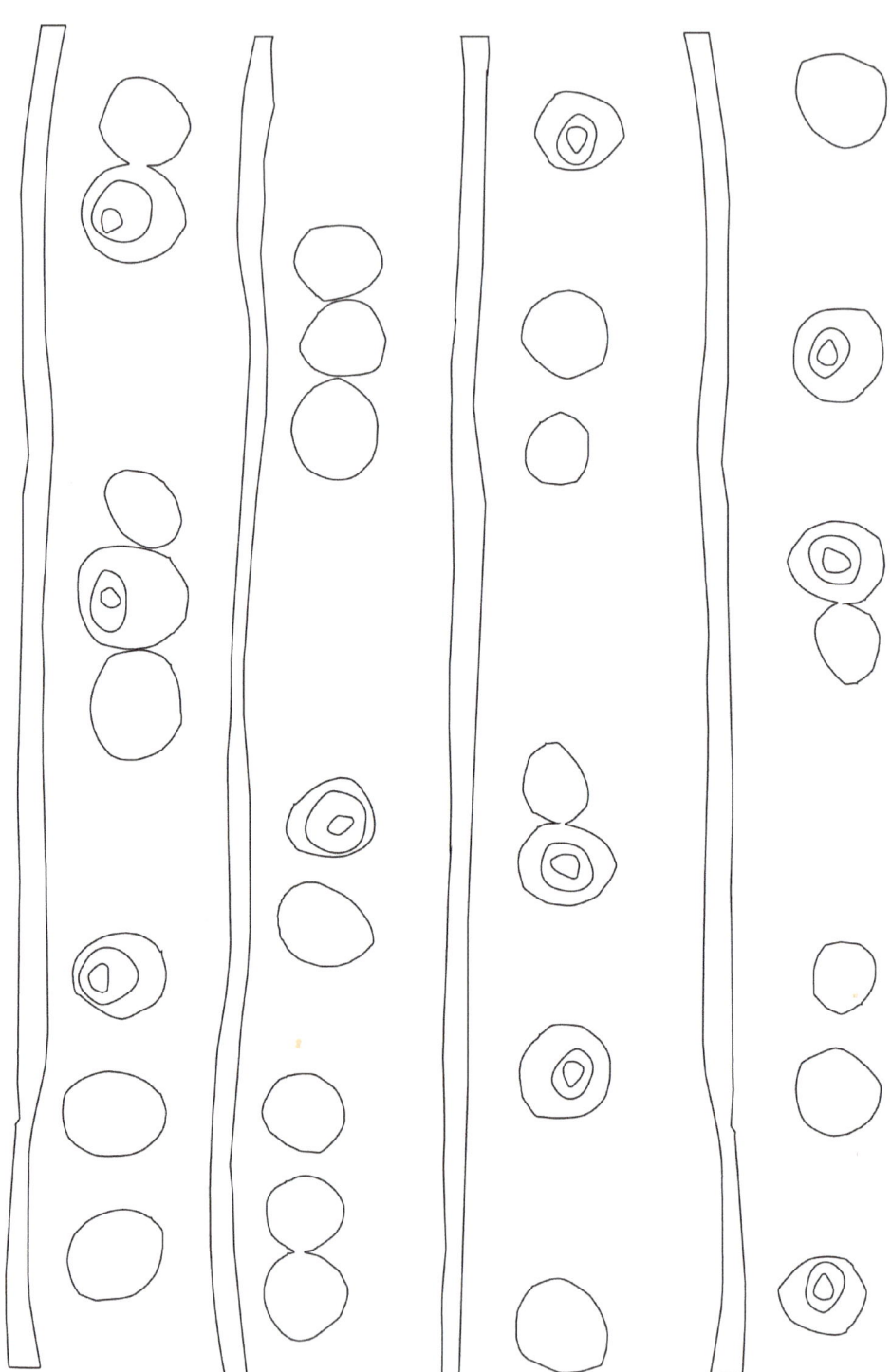

Color to calm your mind and stop overthinking

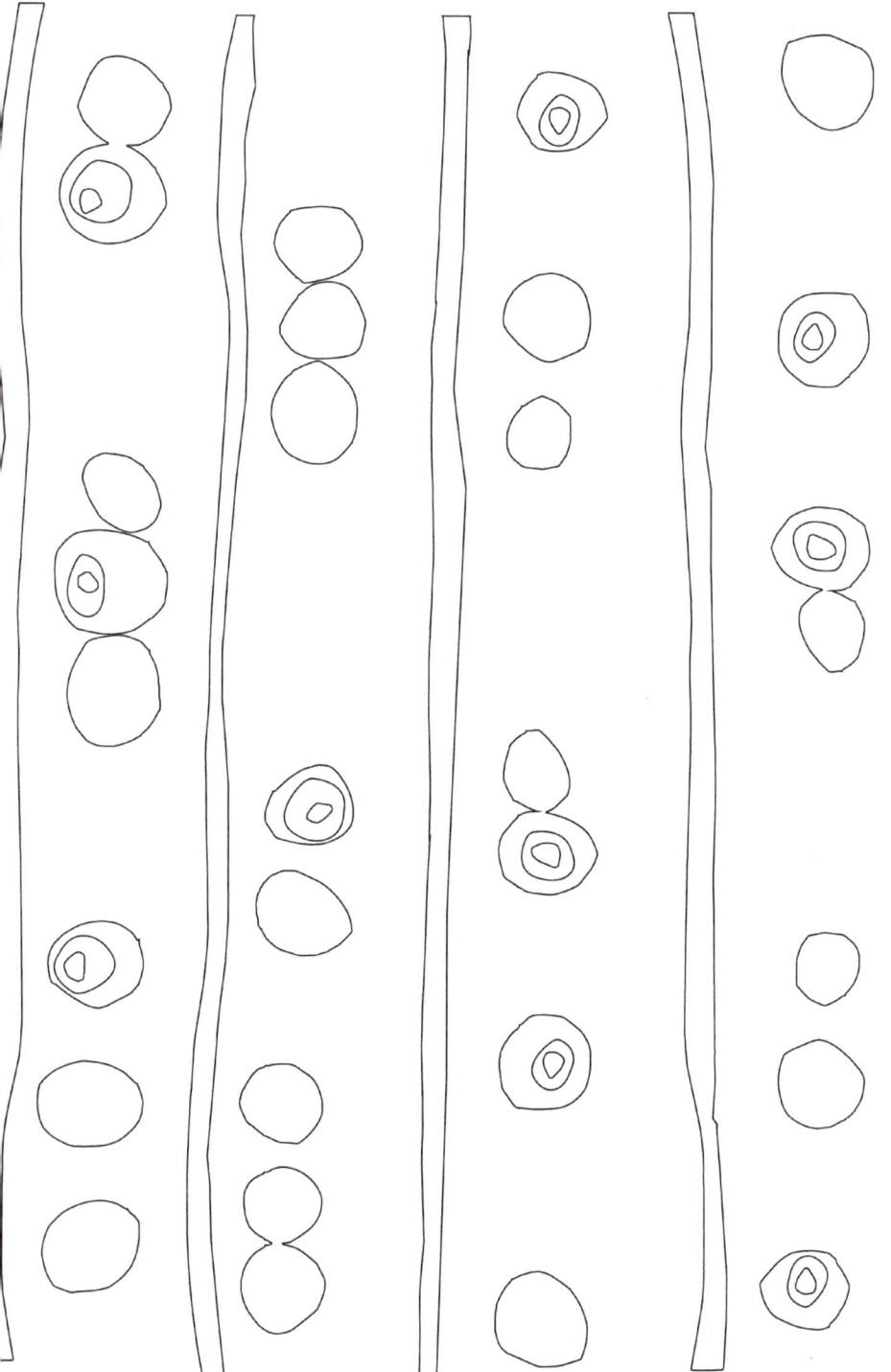

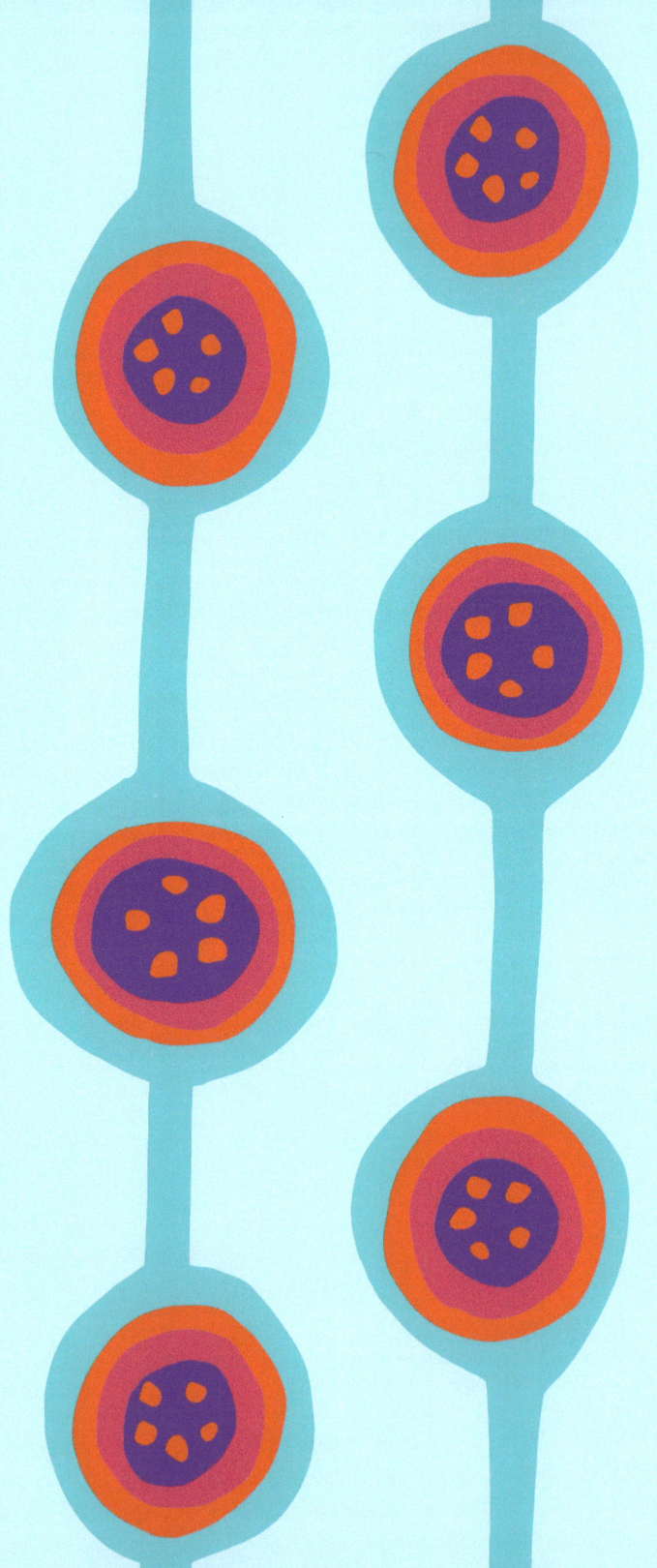

SUMMER

NURTURING YOUR RELATIONSHIPS

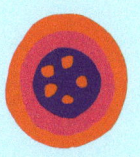

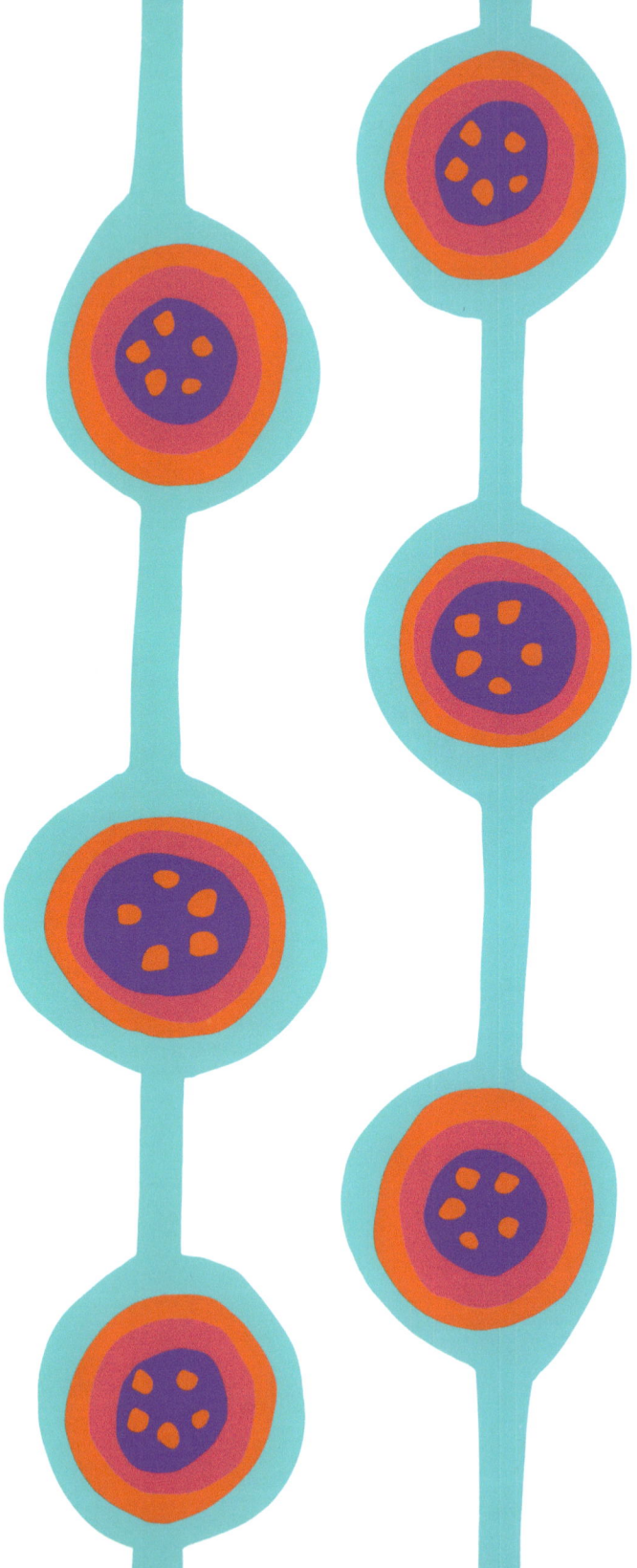

Nurturing Your Relationships

Welcome to summer, where the seeds you planted in spring are starting to sprout, and the warmth of the season invites growth and connection. After delving inward during the previous sections, it's time to turn your attention outward and focus on the people in your life: your friends, family, and community.

Reflect on your relationships. How do they make you feel? Do they support the person you want to become and your goals? Consider whether they will uplift you or hold you back.

If you find some relationships don't align with your path, you'll explore how to change them or let them go. This may involve communicating your needs differently, setting healthy boundaries, or even reevaluating the nature of the relationship.

You'll also think about how you can find new connections that resonate with your new self, through shared interests, values, or goals. You'll seek out individuals who both inspire you and support you.

Assessing your inner circle

THE FIRST STEP is to look at your family, partner, and group of friends, those you hang out with and talk to every day and see if they truly support you. How do you figure that out? Below are a few questions to help you think about them. As you answer the questions, pay attention to how your body feels. Often the body knows the truth before the mind.

If you realize there are people in your life who don't make you feel good after exploring these questions, check out the sections on communication and boundaries later in this section to learn how to improve or let go of these relationships.

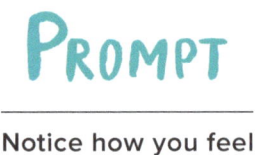

PROMPT

Notice how you feel

What qualities make you feel safe and peaceful around others?

_____

_____

FRIENDS

Think about your closest friends. How do you genuinely feel about them? What sensations arise in your body when you're around them?

_____

_____

_____

PARTNER

If you have a partner, think about how you feel when things are going well between you. Notice the sensations in your body during good times. Then, consider how you feel during disagreements or arguments.

_____

_____

_____

FAMILY

Reflect on your family. How do you feel when you're around them? How does it feel in your body when you're with them? While you can't choose your family, you can prioritize self-care and learn strategies for interacting with them in a way that preserves your emotional well-being.

_____

_____

_____

ACTION STEP   Reconnect with a friend

Think of someone who makes you feel safe and peaceful but haven't talked to recently. Reach out to them via text, phone call, or an e-mail to reconnect. If they're living in a different time zone, schedule a Zoom meet or use an app like Marco Polo for video messages. Remember, nurturing any relationship takes effort, so it's worth investing your time and energy into it.

Assessing your broader community

YOUR WIDER COMMUNITY is surprisingly important to your well-being, even more than you may realize. In fact, according to a recent Harvard longevity study, strong social relationships were found to be the biggest predictor of happiness and health in old age. If you feel disconnected from your community, now is the time to start rebuilding your relationships.

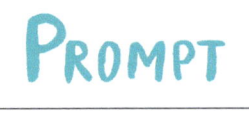

Your ideal community

Describe the personal characteristics you value in people within your ideal community.

_____

_____

_____

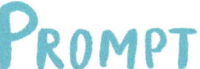

Reflecting on your communities

List the communities you currently belong to (like school, work, clubs, and other groups). Then, consider what steps you can take to foster deeper connections within one or two.

_____

_____

_____

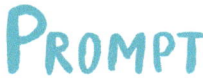

PROMPT

Exploring new communities

Think about new communities you could join, such as school clubs, local committees, book clubs, dance classes, singing groups, church groups, etc. Get creative and think outside the box. You can do a quick Google search or browse local Facebook groups for new ideas. Write down all your ideas here.

_____

_____

_____

_____

_____

ACTION STEP   Connect to new communities

Mark one or two of the new groups you identified with a star to indicate your interest in learning more about them. Write down the time and date of their next meeting, then reach out to the group administrator or join their mailing list. Commit to attending their next meeting. Remember, apart from the time commitment, there's very little to lose and potentially a lot to gain. If this step feels uncomfortable, that's okay. Embrace the challenge and give yourself credit for strengthening your ability to try new things.

Protecting your time and energy with boundaries

SETTING BOUNDARIES to protect your time and energy is essential for your overall well-being. Boundaries act as guidelines that safeguard your physical and emotional health. Every time you decide whether to say "no" to someone's request, you're establishing a boundary. It can be challenging to set and maintain boundaries, especially if you were taught from a young age that your needs aren't as important as others. Yet, prioritizing your own needs is crucial. **Learning to protect yourself—your time, emotions, and personal space—is a skill that takes a lot of practice.**

Saying "yes" to fulfill someone else's happiness while ignoring your own needs can lead to feelings of resentment. Resentment is a subtle form of anger towards another person that slowly builds. Although you may think you're helping by prioritizing their needs and telling them what you think they want to hear, you're ultimately harming the relationship by being inauthentic about your own needs. Over time, this can significantly deteriorate the quality of your relationship. If this pattern sounds familiar, you're not alone. It often stems from childhood messages that have taught you, "My feelings don't matter." If you struggle with this, consider revisiting the section on positive affirmations and crafting one that clearly states that your needs matter.

How others respond to boundaries

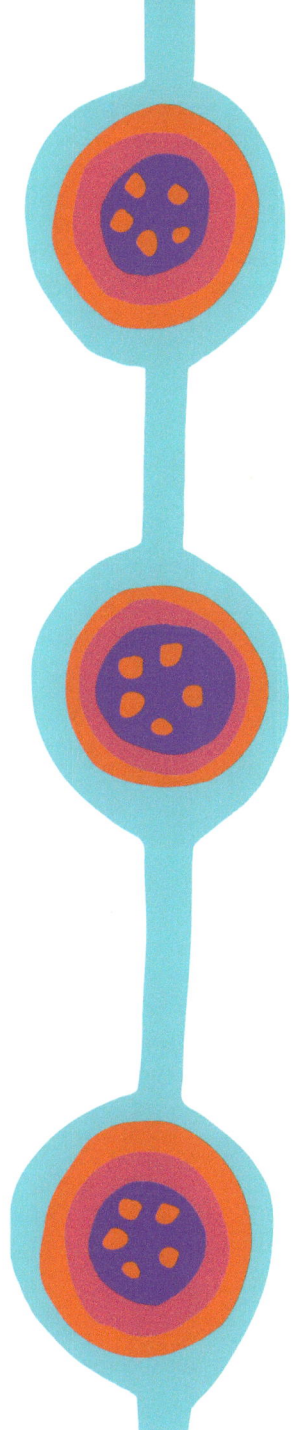

SOME PEOPLE WILL RESPECT and appreciate your boundaries, valuing your clarity regarding your needs. Unfortunately, there are many, particularly those struggling with low self-worth, that may react poorly. For them, hearing a "no" can be challenging, especially if they haven't learned to manage their own emotions, possibly due to childhood messages. They may have learned to expect others to prioritize their needs over their own. Consequently, they might respond with anger or disappointment when faced with a clear boundary.

Despite the discomfort of dealing with adverse reactions, it's essential to maintain your boundaries. Your emotional well-being is your responsibility; you don't need to sacrifice it for others.

If someone's reaction unsettles you, revisit **Stage 1: Winter** and the Emotionally Expressive Journaling exercise to help you deal with difficult emotions. When you notice yourself feeling intensely, take a moment to acknowledge the emotion by saying to yourself, "I notice that I'm feeling _____". Next, BREATHE. Remember, emotions are temporary. It's your thoughts about them that make them stick around longer.

Your emotional well-being is your responsibility; you don't need to sacrifice it for others.

Four steps to set a boundary

A SIMPLE WAY TO REMEMBER how to set a boundary is to use the acronym: STOP. You can remember this because it describes precisely what boundaries do: they stop you from investing your time and energy into people and activities that don't benefit your well-being. Learning to establish clear boundaries is a crucial step in your journey towards change—it allows you to prioritize what best serves your long-term well-being.

STOP to set a boundary:

S   Stop and breathe

T   Tap into your needs

O   Open up direct communication

P   Prioritize yourself

With practice, these steps can become second nature.

Stop and breathe.

When you pause before responding to someone's request for your time or energy, it creates space for your body's intuition (which often knows what's best for you before your mind does) to guide you towards an authentic "yes" or "no."

An authentic "yes" will feel good in your body: you may experience a sense of lightness, centeredness, or a release in your chest or shoulders. Conversely, if you notice tightness in your stomach, chest, or shoulders or experience feelings of discomfort when saying "yes," listen to your body's wisdom! Your choice may not align with your authentic self and could lead to future feelings of resentment.

If you're having trouble deciding whether it's a "yes" or a "no," try the following breathing exercise to feel more grounded.

Five Senses Practice

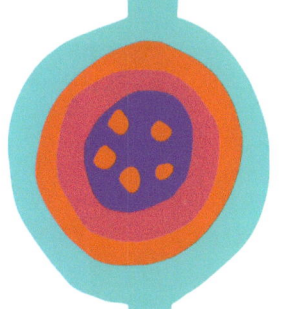

FIRST BREATH: ENVIRONMENT

Breathe in and look around, reminding yourself that you're safe right now.

As you exhale, release any feelings of fear or worry about your external environment.

SECOND BREATH: SOUNDS

Breathe in, close your eyes, and listen carefully to all the sounds around you.

As you exhale, let go of any tension or unease caused by external noises.

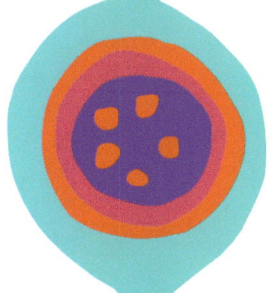

THIRD BREATH: PHYSICAL

Breathe in and notice the sensations between your body and what's supporting it.

As you exhale, release any resistance to this physical contact.

FOURTH BREATH: SCENTS

Breathe in and notice all the different smells around you.

As you exhale, allow yourself to be okay with whatever scents you encounter.

FIFTH BREATH: TASTE

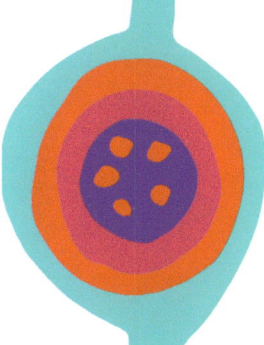

Breathe in and pay attention to any tastes in your mouth.

As you exhale, let yourself be okay with whatever flavors you notice.

With your final inhale, open your eyes and take in your surroundings.

As you exhale, focus on being fully present in the moment.

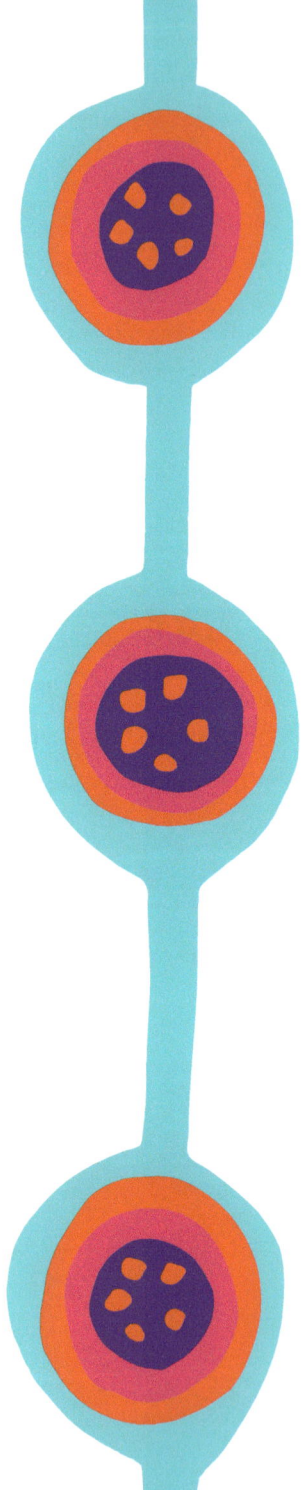

Tap into your needs

Your first instinct may be to say "yes" even when it conflicts with your own needs, especially if you were raised to prioritize others' needs over your own. However, your needs are just as important as those around you. If you're unsure about how you feel after taking a moment, give yourself additional time by saying, "Let me check my calendar, and I'll get back to you," or "I need to think about it." You don't have to give them an immediate answer.

Open up direct communication

How you choose to communicate a boundary will impact its likelihood of success and whether the person reacts defensively or angrily or hears and respects it. Assertive communication, which is direct, intentional, and value-centered, creates understanding. It requires you to take personal responsibility by focusing on yourself and your needs rather than blame the other person.

In the context of communicating a boundary, open communication includes using "I feel" statements rather than statements that address the other person directly (i.e., using the word "you") if and when you feel the need to explain your boundary, as is often the case with someone close to you.

An example: A friend asks you to volunteer for a school event, but you already feel overwhelmed with work and other responsibilities. In response to the request, you might say, "I can't help with the upcoming project. I'm feeling (insert an emotion) because I have already overcommitted myself and have too many responsibilities."

Prioritize yourself

If someone reacts negatively—with anger, disappointment, guilt, or mockery—it can be hurtful. If it happens with someone close to you, try responding directly. Say, "I'm feeling overwhelmed. Let's discuss this when we're both calm," and then step away. Remind yourself silently, "My needs matter just as much as theirs." Remember, it's not your responsibility to manage their emotions; that's up to them. Your job is to take care of yourself. So offer yourself some self-care—take a walk, practice deep breathing or a guided meditation, reach out to a friend, treat yourself to fresh flowers, journal, or practice self-compassion.

Assertive communication, which is direct, intentional, and value-centered, creates understanding.

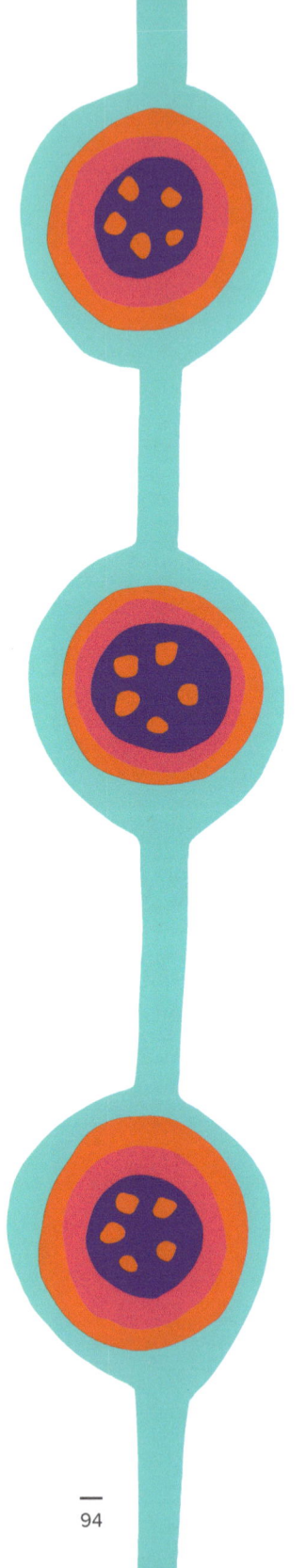

Acts of kindness

CONNECTING WITH OTHERS through acts of kindness, even for those you may not feel close to or agree with, can have remarkable benefits on your emotional and physical well-being and can also uplift others. Displaying kindness may only take a few seconds but can be a profound gift to someone going through a difficult time. A genuine smile directed at someone who appears to be struggling can make a big difference because you never truly know what challenges others are facing. These simple acts not only benefit those around you but also boost your own happiness. Studies show practicing kindness leads to higher levels of well-being.

ACTION STEP Practicing kindness

Choose three acts of kindness and follow through with them.

PROMPT

Exploring kindness towards others

Consider potential acts of kindness. For instance, if a friend seems down, perhaps give them a call to check in. If you receive an e-mail requesting meals for a sick neighbor, sign up to offer your support. Alternatively, if you notice a parent struggling with their children at the store, make eye contact and offer them a sympathetic smile. Brainstorm more acts of kindness and jot them down here.

Finding compassion

PRACTICING COMPASSION can be a powerful tool for connecting with others. By cultivating compassion, you come to understand that everyone faces difficult times and experiences their share of suffering. This understanding can lead to a sense of peace, even in the face of those who may have caused you pain. However, it's essential to remember that cultivating compassion is primarily for your own well-being rather than solely for the benefit of others. It doesn't mean you should tolerate disrespect or allow boundaries to be crossed. Instead, it's about finding your own peace and healing.

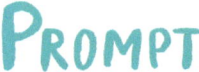

PROMPT

Compassion for strangers

Recall someone random you encountered yesterday, such as the cashier at the grocery store or a stranger on the bus. What do you remember about their face or demeanor? Consider what might be happening in their life. What could they be thinking about or struggling with?

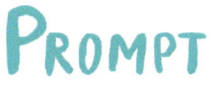

PROMPT

Shared struggles

Think about how people worldwide, regardless of race, nationality, or wealth level, face similar emotional challenges. Write about common ways people collectively endure suffering?

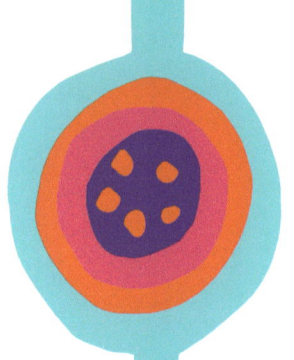

Take time to listen to this guided meditation that will help you feel compassion for people on a more global level.

The gift of forgiveness

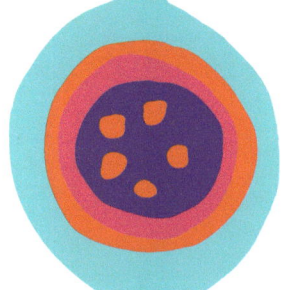

You may have individuals in your life, whether close to you or more distant, who have caused you pain. Perhaps they crossed emotional boundaries or hurt you in some way. Holding onto anger can drain your energy and impact your mental and physical well-being. Consider that you only have a limited amount of daily energy to focus on building the positive life you want. Allowing anger to consume a significant portion hurts your ability to create change. Don't give those who hurt you the power to control your life. But how do you release that anger?

Allowing anger to consume a significant portion of your energy hurts your ability to create change.

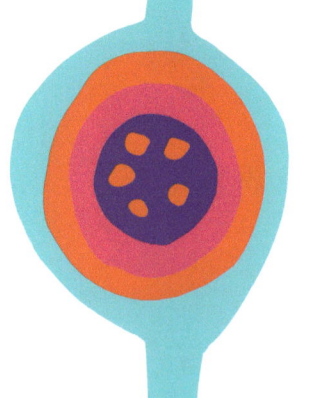

PROMPT

Compassion and forgiveness

Close your eyes, take a deep breath, and think of someone who has emotionally hurt you. Start small, recalling a time when someone hurt your feelings, rather than a person who has deeply emotionally wounded you. You can practice this exercise again, gradually working your way up to those who have hurt you deeply.

Hold that person in your mind. Then, remember the earlier exercise where you thought about the collective struggles of all people. Think about how this person may have experienced suffering in their own life. You don't need to know the specifics of their hardships—this is about imagining. Picture them as a child, facing challenges and difficulties.

If this exercise feels too difficult, return to **Stage 1: Winter** and revisit the Emotionally Expressive Journaling steps. Write about this story and how this person hurt you, explore the emotions it brings up, and then do the meditation where you feel those emotions in your body. Afterward, return here and see if you can find a little more space to cultivate compassion and empathy for the person. If not, that's okay too. **Healing takes time and doesn't follow a fixed schedule.** Give yourself the time and space you need, and then come back here to try again.

Remember, this exercise is for your own benefit. The goal isn't to welcome the person back into your life; they may not deserve a place there. People need to earn the right to occupy your emotional space. The purpose here is to find some peace when you think about them so your emotional and physical health isn't damaged by the toxicity of anger, hurting your chances of moving forward towards positive change.

PROMPT

Compassion and forgiveness (continued)

Think of someone who has emotionally hurt you.

Write about how this person may have experienced suffering in their own life.

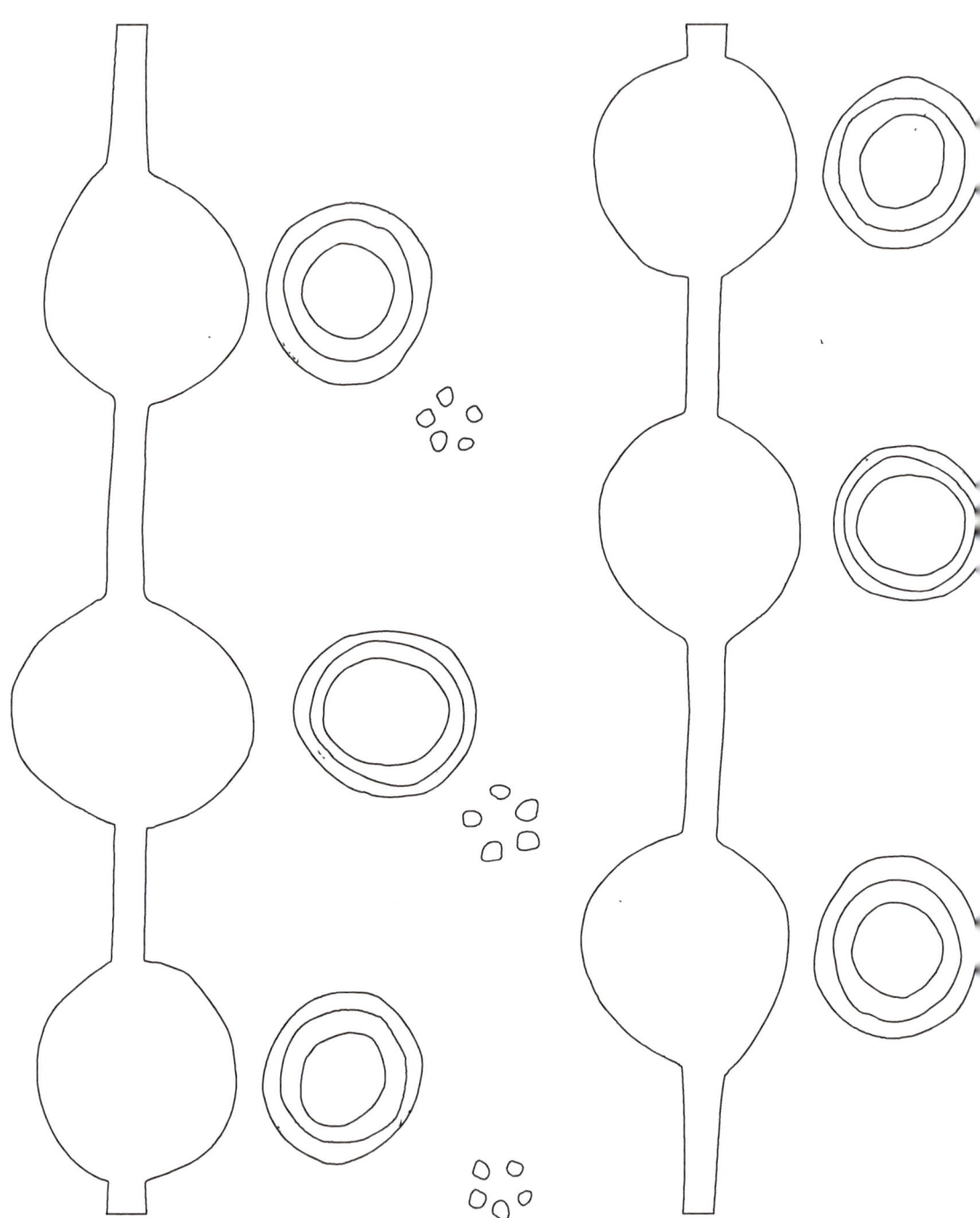

Color to calm your mind and stop overthinking

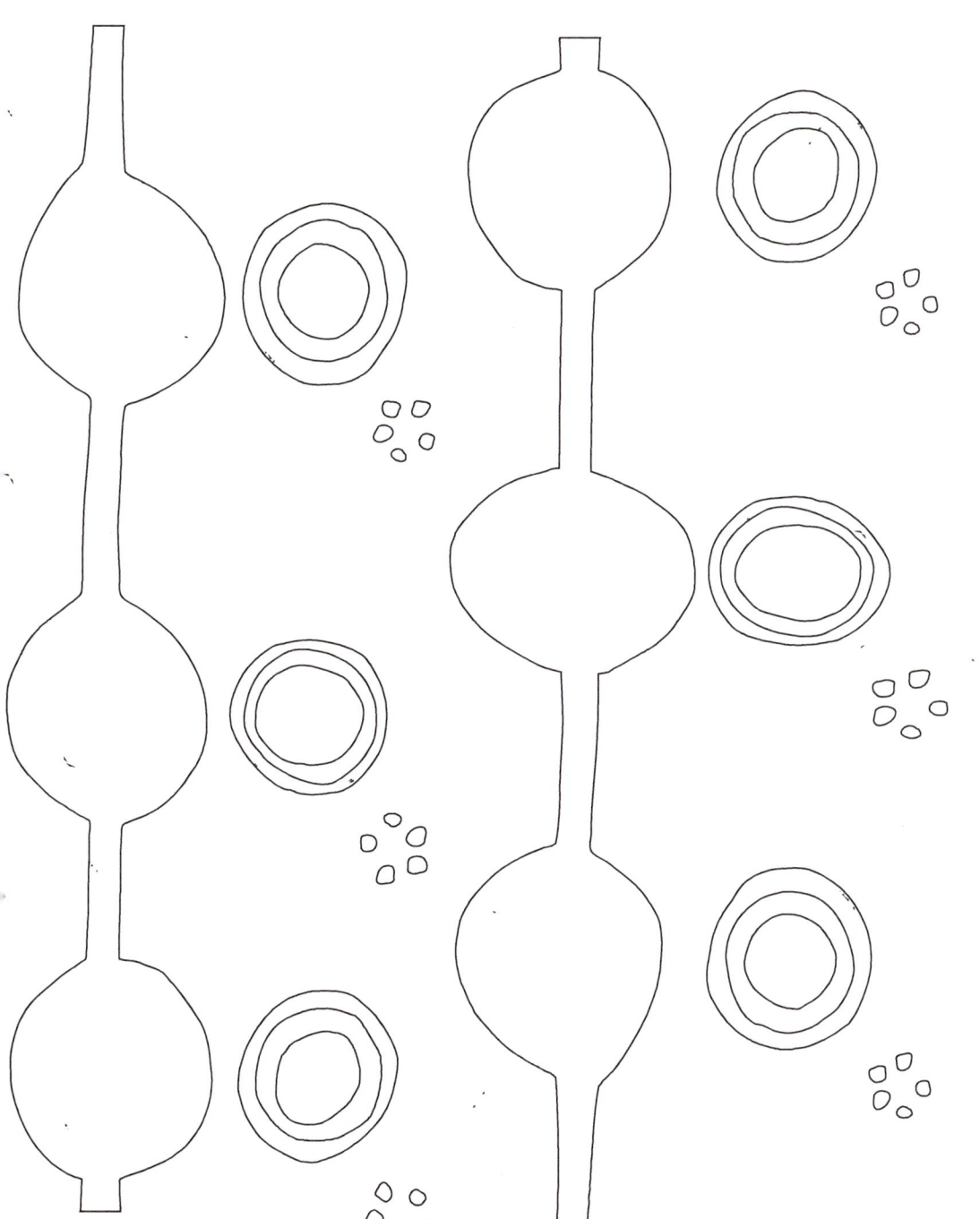

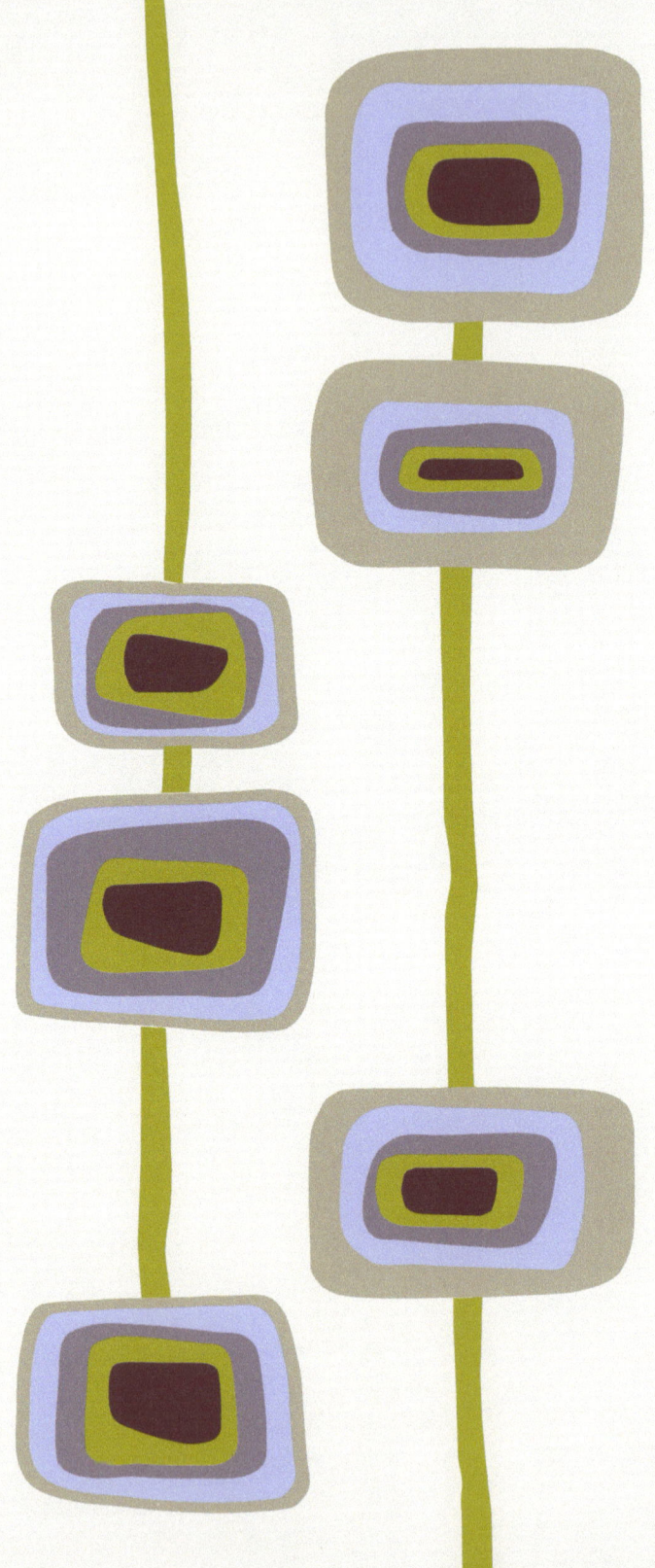

AUTUMN

SAVORING THE GOOD AROUND YOU

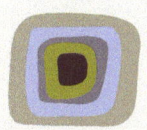

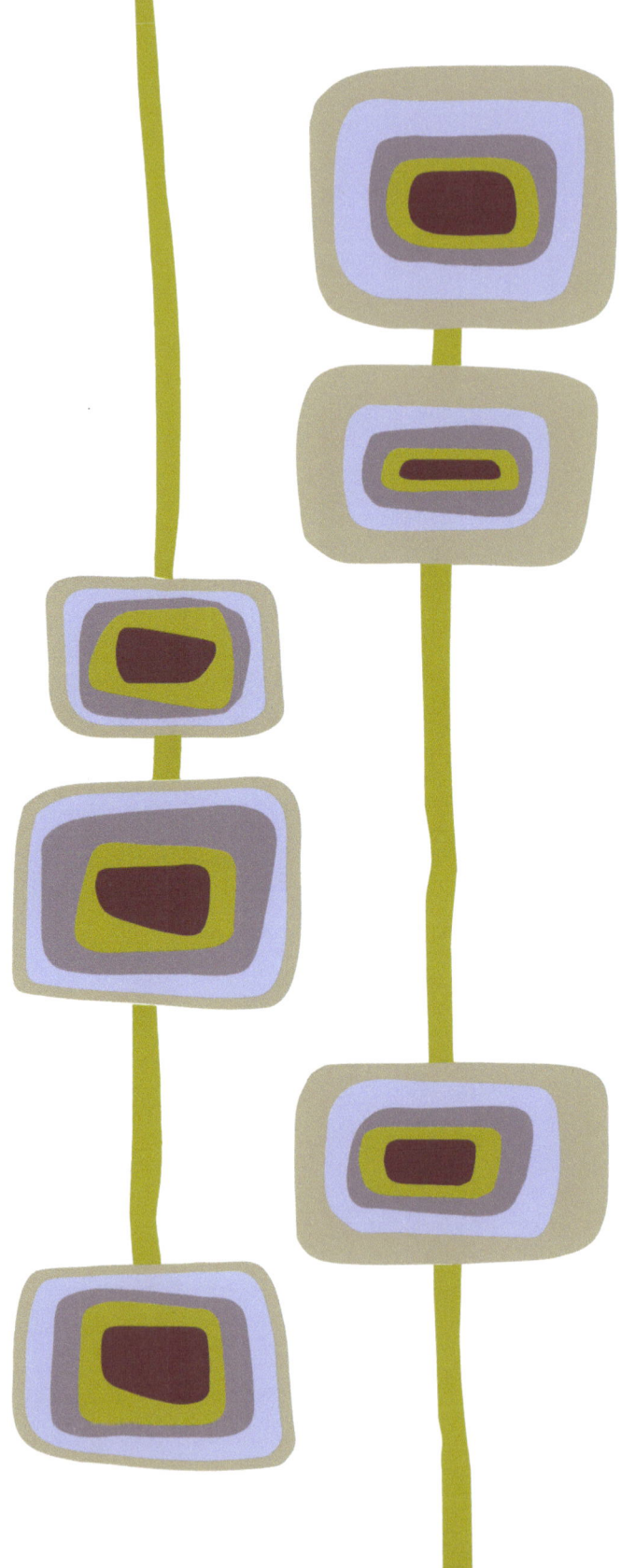

Savoring the Good Around You

You've made it to harvest season! A time to reap the benefits of your perseverance, hard work, and dedication. Take stock of the good in your life and appreciate the abundance that surrounds you. It's a season of celebration, to take time to congratulate yourself on your accomplishments and the work you've done. Look around you: your life may look slightly different now (or perhaps your mindset has changed?). There is a multitude of abundance that surrounds you, and it's time to celebrate the good that exists in your life. As you look around, do you see any blooms from the seeds you planted back in **Stage 2: Spring**?

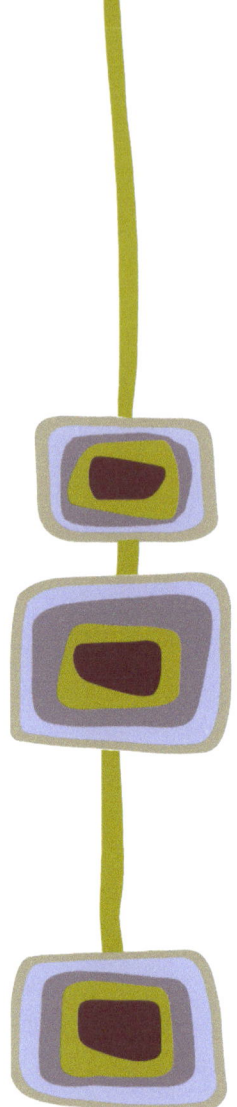

In this section, you will hone your thoughts to find the positives around you. When you're in the midst of change, it's easy to get bogged down in the grind required to forge a new path and lose sight of the positives. The gift of a gratitude practice is that it trains your mind to notice the good in your life, even when you aren't naturally seeing it. As you focus your thoughts on the positives, even the smallest moments, something amazing happens—it becomes easier to find more as the thoughts begin to multiply and new thought pathways become deepened. **The more you focus your thoughts on the good, the more you will experience naturally occurring positive thoughts.** Focusing on what's going well is a crucial step on your pathway to fostering a changed life.

Practicing gratitude

Think of something uplifting from today—a small moment—and hold the sensation in your mind for 20 seconds. How do you feel after? Do you notice a sense of lightness, warmth, calm, or relaxation?

Now, think of something negative from your day. It could be a minor annoyance like someone cutting you off in traffic or an irritating behavior by someone close to you. What do you feel now? Does it feel different?

From this simple exercise, you will find that your focus can influence your emotional state. Positive thoughts make you feel better, while negative ones bring you down. If you want more feelings of contentment, then you have to choose to focus on the positives, and the best way to get started is with a daily gratitude practice.

PROMPT

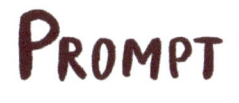

30 days of gratitude

Every night, before you go to bed, take a moment to jot down three positive experiences or thoughts from your day. They can be as small as feeling the warmth of a cup of coffee or tea in your hands, admiring the colors of leaves on trees, or simply enjoying the quiet of the night. You can also include situations or people in your life that bring you joy, like spending time with a child, sibling, friend, parent, or partner, landing a new job, feeling grateful for your home, or doing well on a test. There's no right or wrong way to practice gratitude—just focus on the good things, big or small.

For the next 30 days, write down three positive moments from your day.

DAY 1

1. _____

2. _____

3. _____

DAY 2

1. _____

2. _____

3. _____

DAY 3

1. _____

2. _____

3. _____

DAY 4

1. _____

2. _____

3. _____

DAY 5

1. _____

2. _____

3. _____

DAY 6

1. _____

2. _____

3. _____

DAY 7

1. _____

2. _____

3. _____

DAY 8

1. _____

2. _____

3. _____

DAY 9

1. _____

2. _____

3. _____

DAY 10

1. _____

2. _____

3. _____

DAY 11

1. _____

2. _____

3. _____

DAY 12

1. _____

2. _____

3. _____

DAY 13

1. _____

2. _____

3. _____

DAY 14

1. _____

2. _____

3. _____

DAY 15

1. _____

2. _____

3. _____

DAY 16

1. _____

2. _____

3. _____

DAY 17

1. _____

2. _____

3. _____

DAY 18

1. _____

2. _____

3. _____

DAY 19

1. _____

2. _____

3. _____

DAY 20

1. _____

2. _____

3. _____

DAY 21

1. _____

2. _____

3. _____

DAY 22

1. _____

2. _____

3. _____

DAY 23

1. _____

2. _____

3. _____

DAY 24

1. _____

2. _____

3. _____

DAY 25

1. _____

2. _____

3. _____

DAY 26

1. _____

2. _____

3. _____

DAY 27

1. _____

2. _____

3. _____

DAY 28

1. _____

2. _____

3. _____

DAY 29

1. _____

2. _____

3. _____

DAY 30

1. _____

2. _____

3. _____

BONUS DAY

1. _____

2. _____

3. _____

PROMPT

Reflect on your gratitude journey

As you come to the end of your 30-day gratitude practice,
consider how your perspective has shifted and what
you've learned about yourself and the world around you.

Moving forward, how do you plan to incorporate
gratitude into your daily routine?

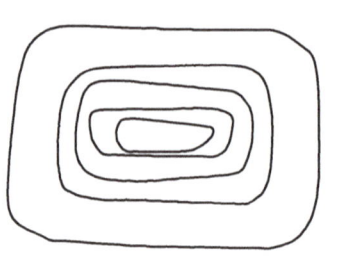

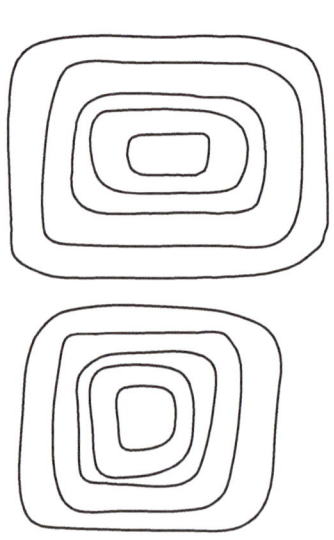

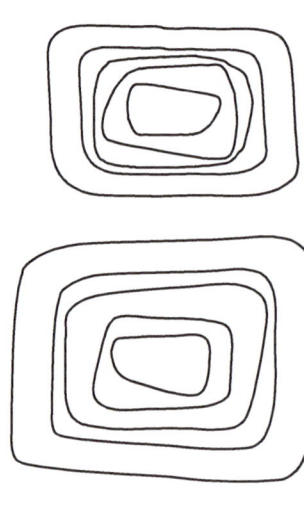

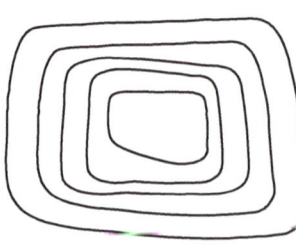

Color to calm your mind and stop overthinking

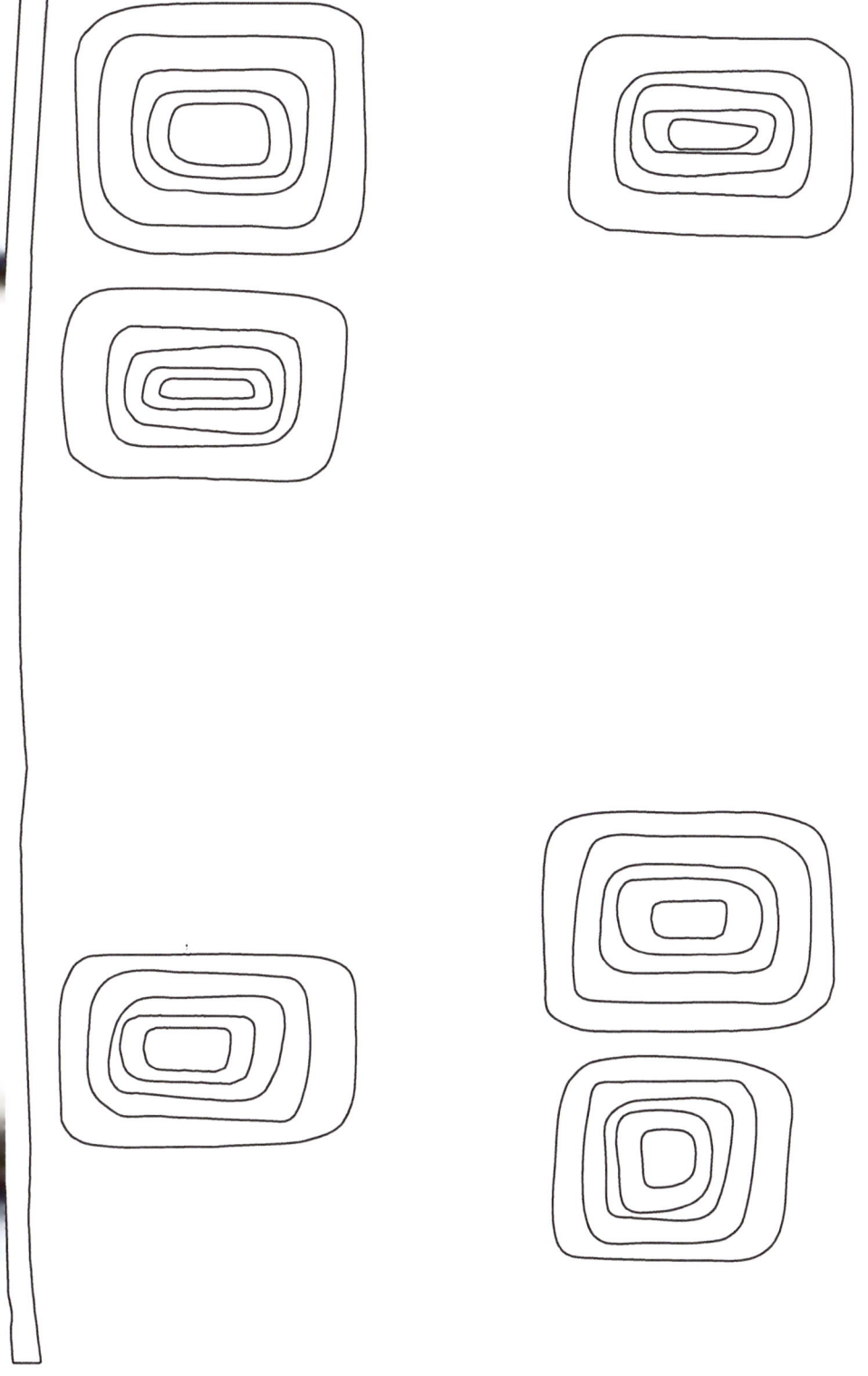

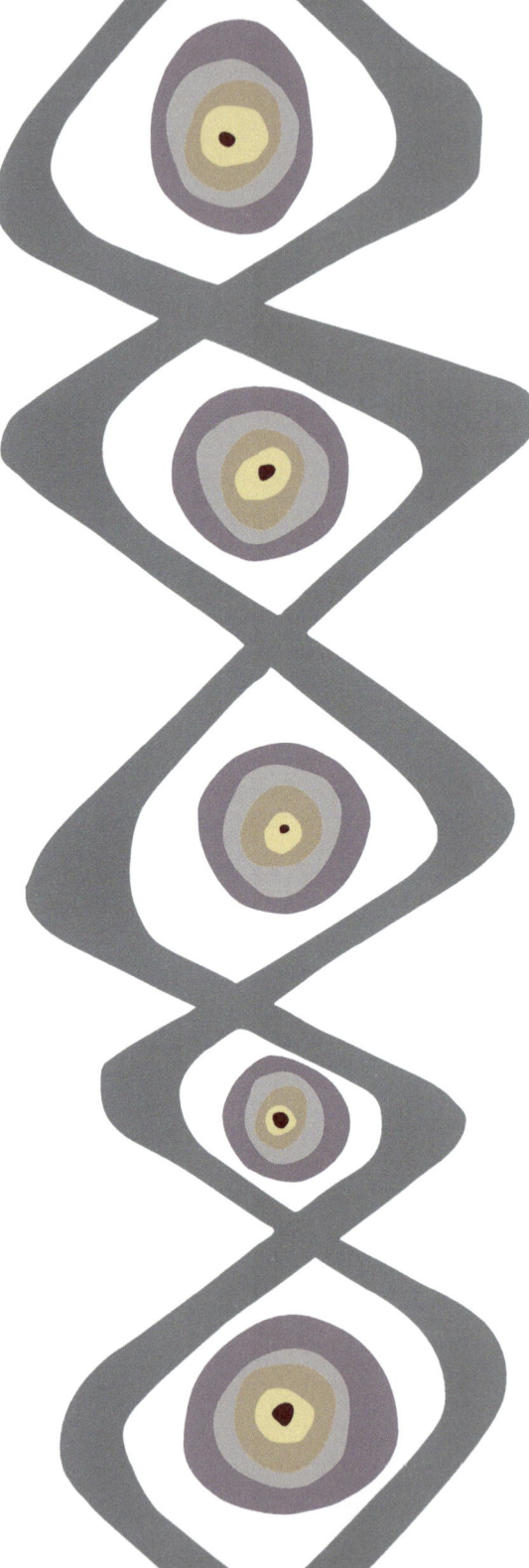

Final Reflections

You've changed since starting this journey and have altered the course of your path. You know yourself better now, and you're learning to view your thoughts as just thoughts, giving you newfound freedom in how you respond to situations. You've gained insight into what's not working in your life and identified areas for change, perhaps even witnessing tangible shifts. Whether showing yourself compassion, challenging limiting beliefs, or setting boundaries to protect your well-being, you now possess invaluable tools for navigating life's inevitable changes.

Which insights or lessons from BREATHE resonated most deeply with you?

What steps will you take to integrate them into your daily life?

Remember, progress is made one step at a time. Just as you train your body, your mind also requires ongoing attention. Make time for self-care, whether it's through meditation, extending compassion to yourself, revisiting the Ideal Day Exercise when things feel out of alignment, doing a quick satisfaction assessment on the Wheel of Life, or practicing boundaries. **These tools are here for you whenever you need them.**

About

BREATHE was created by Kate Simpson. The idea for this journal came from watching her teenagers and their friends struggle to find helpful resources during the tough days of COVID. It was created with input from Ray Baskerville, who reviewed and contributed valuable content and recorded its beautiful, guided meditations. BREATHE builds on the work found in *Take Two: A Journal for New Beginnings*, a guided journal published by Chronicle Books in 2020 and created collaboratively by Kate, Kari Herer, and Ellen Watson Cady.

Kate Simpson: Author

Kate is the Co-Author of *Take Two: A Journal for New Beginnings*, which helps people build emotional resilience. She is also the Co-Founder and Head of Outreach for ValuesAdvisor, a nonprofit platform that connects investors to financial advisors to align their investments with their values. Kate received a B.A. in English literature from Boston College and a Master's degree in education from Stanford University. She resides in Maine with her husband and three children.

Ray Baskerville: Meditation Creator

Ray has been a practicing meditator for over 30 years and author of several books on meditation and mindfulness as healing and therapeutic practices. Ray is a certified hypnotherapist, holds a Master's Degree in mindfulness-based psychotherapy, is currently completing a Doctorate in clinical psychology, and has received training in EMDR. He currently works as an attachment-focused therapist and transpersonal coach in Maui, Hawaii, where he resides with his family. **raybaskerville.com**

Joellen McCosh: Artist

Joellen is the owner of olive + you, a small interior wall decor company based in Yarmouth, Maine. Her work focuses on the interaction between emotions, color, shape, and space in our interior and exterior worlds. She holds a B.S. in biology with a minor in art from Allegheny College and a Master's degree in speech-language pathology from Purdue University. Joellen resides in Maine with her husband and two children. **oliveandyou.com**

Diane Dempsey Murray: Designer

Diane is an art director and visual designer experienced at transforming ideas into captivating visuals. Specializing in concept development, art direction and visual design, she bring brands to life across marketing, social campaigns, and editorial projects for print and digital media. **ddmurray.com**

Kari Herer: Design Consultant

Kari is a Maine-based professional photographer and printmaker and has been a featured artist on Etsy, *Design*Sponge*, and *Click Magazine* and collaborated with Anthropologie, IKEA, *Martha Stewart Weddings*, and Restoration Hardware. She conducts photography workshops around the U.S. **kariherer.com**

Ellen Watson Cady: Editor

Ellen is the Co-Author of *Take Two: A Journal for New Beginnings*. She also manages the social media strategy for a nonprofit and is a trained yoga teacher, a freelance writer, and a mom to two daughters. As a writer and mother, she's inspired daily by the sights and sounds of the outdoors and its natural beauty, taking her children on as many adventures as she can muster.

Anna Mantzaris: Editor

Anna is a San Francisco-based writer and editor. She has worked with publishing, nonprofit, and advertising clients. She teaches writing in the M.F.A. program at Bay Path University. **annamantzaris.net**

Author's Note

While I may have compiled these practices into this particular format, the ideas and concepts come from many teachers, researchers, and psychologists, and I can't take credit for them. I offer gratitude to each and every one of them who has shared their research and ideas freely.

Check out BREATHE's Resource Page for suggested books and podcasts or to learn more about the academic research behind the practices offered here.

breathe-journal.com/resources

Copyright: BREATHE: A Guided Journal

ISBN: 979-8-218-43298-0

www.ingramcontent.com/pod-product-compliance
Lightning Source LLC
Chambersburg PA
CBHW040851120626.
46547CB00006B/570